Ten years ago, it had been so frequent Maya had almost come to expect it.

She'd see someone in a crowded street, or getting on a plane, or among the audience at a conference that would remind her of Eli—the same height or with the same dark hair or that wide smile, perhaps, and she'd quicken her pace or simply stare at them until it became quite clear that it wasn't him. And then she'd have to cope with a wave of heartbreak that was an actual, physical pain.

But...*here*...?

On a small, South Pacific Island right on the outskirts of the Fijian archipelago?

A *private* island?

It wasn't possible.

Except...it kind of was, if you took into account that Reki Island was about to host a camp for children with complex medical needs who couldn't attend the usual holiday camps for kids. And that qualified volunteers, like Maya, came from all over the world to take part in the ten days that were life-changing for the children who were lucky enough to get chosen to come here.

And that Eli Peters was still—as far as Maya knew, anyway—a doctor.

Dear Reader,

Living at the bottom of the world in New Zealand, I've been lucky enough to spend time on quite a few Pacific Islands, and I absolutely love the romance of palm-fringed, white-sanded beaches and gorgeous sunsets. It's the perfect setting for a story where my characters, Eli and Maya, unexpectedly meet each other again after many years apart.

Throw in a camp for medically fragile children with their own stories that will tug at your heartstrings, a wild storm and a hair-raising rescue or two, and it became a joy to write.

Happy reading!

With love,

Alison xxx

PARAMEDIC'S
REUNION IN PARADISE

ALISON ROBERTS

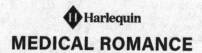

MEDICAL ROMANCE

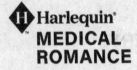

Harlequin®
MEDICAL ROMANCE

Recycling programs
for this product may
not exist in your area.

ISBN-13: 978-1-335-94282-1

Paramedic's Reunion in Paradise

Harlequin Enterprises ULC
22 Adelaide St. West, 41st Floor
Toronto, Ontario M5H 4E3, Canada
www.Harlequin.com

Printed in U.S.A.

Alison Roberts has been lucky enough to live in the South of France for several years recently but is now back in her home country of New Zealand. She is also lucky enough to write for the Harlequin Medical Romance line. A primary school teacher in a former life, she later became a qualified paramedic. She loves to travel and dance, drink champagne, and spend time with her daughter and her friends. Alison Roberts is the author of over one hundred books!

Books by Alison Roberts

Harlequin Medical Romance

A Tale of Two Midwives

Falling for Her Forbidden Flatmate
Miracle Twins to Heal Them

Daredevil Doctors

Forbidden Nights with the Paramedic
Rebel Doctor's Baby Surprise

Morgan Family Medics

Secret Son to Change His Life
How to Rescue the Heart Doctor

Paramedics and Pups

The Italian, His Pup and Me

Healed by a Mistletoe Kiss
Therapy Pup to Heal the Surgeon
City Vet, Country Temptation

Visit the Author Profile page
at Harlequin.com for more titles.

Praise for
Alison Roberts

"The love story is built up slowly but surely with just the right amount of passion and tenderness. This novel will tug at your heartstrings and give you hope in miracles. All romance readers need to grab a copy of this terrific tale ASAP."

—*Harlequin Junkie* on
A Paramedic to Change Her Life

CHAPTER ONE

OH, NO...

Not now.

Please...

Maya Thompson had been heading for the biggest space amongst the resort buildings—the dining room and conference area that made a U shape around the largest swimming pool.

She knew there would be a buffet breakfast laid out and she'd been really looking forward to that first taste of some of her favourite fresh tropical fruit like mangos and pawpaw but she had just lost her appetite completely.

Maybe it was because it hadn't happened for so long that it had caught her unawares. Or maybe it was because this was the last place she would have expected it to happen.

Ten years ago, it had been so frequent Maya had almost come to expect it. She'd see someone in a crowded street, or getting on a plane, or amongst the audience at a conference that would remind her of Eli—the same height or with the same dark hair or that wide smile, perhaps, and she'd quicken her pace or simply stare at them until it became quite clear that it wasn't him. And then she'd have to cope with a wave of heartbreak that was an actual physical pain.

But...*here*...?

On a small South Pacific Island right on the outskirts of the Fijian archipelago?

A *private* island?

It wasn't possible.

Except...it kind of was, if you took into account that Reki Island was about to host a camp for children with complex medical needs who couldn't attend the usual holiday camps for kids and that qualified volunteers, like Maya, came from all over the world to take part in the ten days that were life-changing for the children that were lucky enough to get chosen to come here.

And that Eli Peters was still—as far as Maya knew, anyway—a doctor.

It didn't matter how unlikely it was; in this moment Maya needed a few minutes to herself and she knew exactly where she needed to go. She took a left turn onto a different track that led past a string of round *bures* with thatched roofs that provided individual sleeping and bathroom facilities, and she kept walking until the paved pathways that were designed to cater for wheelchairs or walking aids gave way to soft sand and the occasional coconut that had fallen from the palm trees that lined a perfect crescent of white sand and a lagoon that was still tinged with the pink of a fading sunrise.

Maya took off her white slip-on canvas sneakers and held them in her hand as she walked to where the tiniest waves barely lapped the firmer damp sand. A soft tropical breeze made her curly hair tickle the nape of her neck and she took in a very deep breath and then closed her eyes as she let it out slowly.

Was she going to let an unexpected mental hiccup sabotage something that only happened once a year? Something that Maya looked forward to more than Christmas, New Year celebrations, her birthday or…pretty much everything else put together?

Of course she wasn't.

Reki Island was not only a physical paradise, with its warm sunshine, perfect beaches, lush forests and both sunrises and sunsets that belonged on postcards, it brought together everything that mattered most to Maya. Her job, friendship, children, adventure and…the joy of belonging. Being needed, in fact. This was a place and time where both her profession as a highly trained paramedic and her skills in the leisure activities she loved made her the perfect fit as a volunteer for Reki Island's sought-after camp experience for children with special needs.

'Maya?'

Her eyes flew open and she turned her head sharply but it wasn't a ghost walking towards her from the shadows of the palm trees.

'Mike…' Maya could feel her smile reaching as far as her eyes. 'How good to see you.'

Their hug was full of genuine warmth. Mike might have made it clear years ago that he hoped for more than friendship but that had never been an option and Maya felt completely safe with him. She had encouraged his dream of setting up the camp and hadn't hesitated to become a part of it herself.

'I'm sorry I wasn't still awake when you arrived last night,' Maya said as she stepped back. 'I didn't even hear the chopper landing.'

'I'm sorry I wasn't here to welcome you earlier. I had no intention of getting caught up in a management crisis back in my hospital in the States, but there you go. I knew Team Reki were more than capable of putting the finishing touches on the months of setting up and I promised that nothing was going to stop me getting back in time for the first day of camp. Not when it's our fifth anniversary.'

Mike Davis shaded his eyes against the rising sun as he gazed out towards the reef and he echoed the way Maya had taken a breath and let it out in a sigh. 'I feel like we're established now,' he said. 'This place is exactly what I wanted it to be. And it can grow. The income from the resort is more than enough to fund expansion and we've got waiting lists of kids who are desperate to come. We're going to look at running a second camp very soon.'

'It's an amazing achievement,' Maya said quietly. 'I'm very glad that there are some people in the world who use their wealth to do something this special. You can be very proud of what you've created and how many lives you've changed for the better. Not just for the kids but for their whole families.'

Mike shrugged off the praise. 'I got lucky. It was past time for my family's fortune to do some good in the world. Going to camp was the best thing in my life as a kid, but it would have been so much better if my brother had been able to come as well.'

Maya nodded. She knew the story. Mike's younger brother had been too sick to ever be considered for a summer camp and his death as a teenager had left a scar deep enough to motivate Mike to train as a doctor and become a paediatrician. Wealthy enough to buy a private island with an existing resort, he'd added a state-of-the-art medical facility and then collected a passionate team of medics and other helpers who were prepared to volunteer their time and skills. He'd been the driving force behind creating a unique camp for a very special group of children and young people who were facing serious health challenges.

'How many campers do we have this time?'

'Thirty, if they're all still well enough to make it. We've got volunteers meeting some of them at the airport in Nadi this morning to bring them out to the island, but most have got a carer with them.' He glanced at his watch. 'Breakfast should be done by now. I want to get our briefing out of the way so we can all get ready for a busy day. Coming?'

'Of course. You go ahead, though, Mike. I'll need to get the sand off my feet and put my shoes back on. There's bound to be a dozen people who are waiting to talk to you before the staff meeting begins.'

Mike nodded and was gone with a smile and a wave. Maya stayed where she was for just another breath, watching the island's owner and camp director stride towards the tracks where glimpses of thatched roofs could be seen amongst the lush greenery. Shifting her gaze towards the end of the crescent beach, she could see the rocky outcrop that was the bottom of their very own mountain and out to sea were the tiny islands whose only inhabitants were huge sea turtles and a rainbow of tropical fish.

Maya realised she was still smiling as she turned her back on the view. Moments later, she balanced herself against the trunk of a palm tree as she brushed sand off her feet and then put her shoes back on.

And why wouldn't she be smiling? This was her happy place.

Maya had been a part of this since well before the very first camp. She'd even helped to choose the name of the island. *Reki* meant 'something joyous' in Fijian and it was also part of *ka reki-taki*, which meant 'delight'—the provision of which was exactly what Mike's mission was for the children who came here during the part of the year that the resort was closed to other clients. She'd also been involved in designing the uniform she was wearing that was comfortable and practical, with the sneakers, a pair of navy-blue shorts that had a cuff just above knee level and a white polo shirt that had her name badge on one side and an embroidered 'Star of Life' symbol on the other. She loved the bright red, blunt-pointed star with the white snake wrapped around the staff in its centre that was an internationally recognised badge of qualification for someone in an emergency medical service. She was proud to wear it.

Maya straightened her spine. She was proud of everything about Reki Island and her part in its history and purpose.

The blip of memory of a relationship that had failed in such a hauntingly spectacular fashion was not going to change anything. It was so far in the past now it was irrelevant, anyway.

Just like Eli Peters was.

'Are you listening, Simon?'

'Look at *this*, Dad...'

The young boy was lying on his stomach. Open in front of him on the floor was the information booklet for the Reki Island Children's Camp—a thick volume of laminated pages full of instructions, explanations and photographs. The page Simon was pointing to had children wearing helmets and harnesses, abseiling down what looked like a sheer rock cliff.

'That's so cool,' Simon said. 'I want to sign up to try that.'

'No.' Eli Peters shook his head. 'Sorry, Si, but that's not going to happen.'

'Why not?'

'You know why.'

'But it says in here that the people who take these activities are able to let every child experience them safely within their level of capability.'

That a nine-year-old could read this well gave

Eli a glow of pride but he had to make something very clear.

'We talked about this and you know the rules.
Some things are going to be too dangerous for
you and anything like rock climbing or abseiling are at the top of the list.'

He wasn't about to try and scare Simon by
reminding him that it wouldn't take much of a
bump from some sharp volcanic rock to cause
internal bleeding that could be life-threaten-
ing. And yes, he'd brought Factor VIII and
tranexamic acid himself to boost the medical
supplies they had available here for children with
haemophilia A but...they were in the middle of
the Pacific Ocean and even with a helicopter on
the island and Mike's private jet in Nadi they
were a hell of a long way away from the kind
of hospital Eli would be happy for Simon to be
getting any major surgery done.

'But, *Dad...*'

'No buts,' Eli said firmly. 'Now... I'm about
to go to a staff meeting. Someone should be here
any minute to look after you, okay?'

'I don't need looking after. I'm nearly *ten.*'

'*Bula...*' The cheerful greeting was coming
from the *bure's* veranda. 'I'm Ana. Are you Dr
Peters?'

The young Fijian woman was wearing a bright
pink and white dress and had a matching pink

flower tucked behind her ear. She was also wearing the widest, brightest smile Eli had ever seen. It was impossible not to smile back.

'I am. Come in, Ana. Simon's in here.'

'You're lucky,' Ana told Simon when she saw what he was looking at. 'You're the first one here for camp so there'll be lots of space for you to choose which activities you want to do first when we go over to the big room later.'

Eli caught Simon's gaze. He didn't have to say anything. They'd already been through the huge list of available activities. Simon would be able to go swimming, snorkelling, sailing, kayaking and paddle boarding for water sports. He could go on forest walks and boat trips to see the turtles. He could join in games like balloon tennis and mini golf, and then there were all the art and craft sessions, dance, music and cooking classes, a scavenger hunt and a talent show to take part in. Pony riding had been a major concession on Eli's part but he was assuming that any animal chosen to interact with medically fragile children would be completely safe.

Simon might be scowling back at him but he really couldn't complain about being banned from high impact activities like rock climbing, abseiling or water sliding. The next ten days were probably going to be packed with more excitement than he'd ever had in his life.

Ana looked up at Eli. 'You'll be busy all morning, yes?'

'Yes. There's a staff meeting and then the tour of the medical facilities. I'll get a break a lunchtime, I expect.'

'Don't worry about Simon,' Ana said. 'I will take very good care of him. He can come and help greet all the campers that will start arriving on the boats soon and I'll take him to put his name on the lists for tomorrow's activities.' She smiled at Simon. 'Did you know that there's a huge bonfire tonight? And a barbecue dinner to welcome everybody to Camp Reki. There'll be lots of singing and dancing. And drumming. Can you play the drums, Simon?'

He shook his head.

'Would you like to learn?'

Simon's nod was eager.

'There's a class for that,' Ana said, 'but if we get time I'll take you to meet my little brother, Tevita. He's about your age and he can teach you some drumming today. That way, you could come and help welcome the boats when they arrive.'

'Yes, *please*… Can we go and see him now?'

Simon's eyes were shining and he'd clearly forgotten any resentment about the banned activities. Eli gave Ana a grateful glance as he left. He needed to hurry now and find the way back to where they'd had breakfast to be in time for the staff meeting that everybody involved with the medical side of the camp was required to attend.

It looked as if most of the huge medical team were already gathered by the time Eli reached the space where tables had been cleared away and replaced by rows of chairs. There was a whiteboard at the front of the room and Mike was clearly trying to get his laptop connected to deliver a presentation.

Eli looked around the room, trying to find a spare seat, but people were still moving, leaning over the backs of chairs to shake hands or hug people they obviously knew well. He couldn't tell what chairs were about to be used or who intended to sit beside those already seated. How many of these people had been here before? There was a lot of chatter and laughter going on and for a moment Eli felt as if he didn't belong.

He'd loved social gatherings once, though, hadn't he? Had he shut himself off so much from normal life in recent years that he'd turned into some kind of recluse? He really did feel a bit like the new boy at school at the moment.

Almost...vulnerable?

He hadn't expected quite this many people.

And...

No...

It couldn't be. Could it…?

Eli could feel his brows almost meeting at the top of his nose, in a mix of a downward frown and an upward question. He couldn't see the woman's face because she was at the front of the room but that wild, dark curly hair made him think instantly of Maya.

And the feeling in his gut was just the same as it always had been whenever he thought of her.

That hollow sensation that was all about loss.

Regret.

And okay…maybe there was still a bit of anger somewhere, if he dug deep enough.

Which he wasn't going to do, of course. What would be the point of that?

It was ten years ago, for heaven's sake.

Eli couldn't imagine why his memory had ambushed him quite like this, but it wasn't hard to dismiss. It was, after all… What was the word he was looking for?

Oh, yeah…*irrelevant*.

The hum of conversation in the conference room faded as Mike Davis moved to stand beside the whiteboard, holding a microphone in his hand as he looked at all the people in front of him.

These were the specialist dieticians, psychologists, physios and occupational therapists, paramedics, nurses and doctors that had come here to take care of the special requirements of children with complex medical needs.

'First of all,' he said, 'as the medical director and founder of Camp Reki, I want to welcome you to the island and to extend my heartfelt thanks to you all for giving so much of your time and expertise to this project—without you, none of this would be possible. Many of you have been here before—some have been a vital part of the operation since the very beginning.' He was smiling as he looked straight at Maya, who was sitting at the side of the front row. 'Others are here for the first time, so I want to give you a special welcome.'

There was a wave of applause as Mike lifted a hand in a gesture towards someone who was at the back of the room. Maya turned her head but there were a couple of latecomers moving to empty seats and she couldn't see anyone acknowledging his mention.

'We'll do some introductions later,' Mike continued, 'but let's crack on. We want to get through all the housekeeping stuff and a tour of the facilities before our campers are all here by this afternoon and are coming in for their initial check-ups. I know you've all received information on anyone who's been flagged as needing your particular areas of expertise but I'd like everyone to be familiar with the group as a whole.

You may well be asked to get involved with other children, so we'll run through a quick overview of medical histories for the kids we're expecting this time.'

Mike tapped a key on his laptop and the whiteboard filled with a montage of pictures. One was a child on the back of a pony with a helper on either side to support them. Another was holding up shells they were collecting on a beach. Some were on surfboards or in the sea with snorkels and facemasks on. There were wheelchairs deep in the forest and children in special harnesses on a zipline. The activities portrayed were all different but what every photo had in common was the expression on the faces of the children.

Sheer joy…

'As you know,' he began, 'the children can't come to camp unless they've been given a recent all-clear from their own doctors that they're stable and don't have a condition or potential complications that might endanger the health, safety or emotional well-being of themselves or other campers or any of the staff but, as you also know, accidents or unexpected medical events can happen any time or anywhere and there's no denying that the range of experiences we offer here increases the risk factors, no matter how well we aim to manage them.'

He tapped again and the image changed to one

of a girl with long brown hair who was sitting on a beach, helping to make a sandcastle—holding a bucket despite having no hands.

'This is Hazel,' Mike said. 'Eleven years old and this will be her fourth time at camp. Meningitis as a toddler left her a multiple amputee, losing both hands and feet. She also has some hearing loss, so it helps to make sure she can see your face when you're talking to her. She's medically stable and very independent.'

Independent and as keen as mustard to try anything. Maya had fallen in love with this little girl when she'd been here as an eight-year-old, determined to have a go at the climbing wall with the help of a harness, ropes and Maya dangling behind her. She wouldn't be at all surprised if Hazel intended to try out a real cliff this year.

Mike moved on swiftly through the group of children who, like Hazel, were stable and confident enough to be here without a personal carer. Amongst others, there was Mason, who was a badly scarred burns survivor, and Scarlett, who was currently in remission from her cancer.

Mike was clicking through the case histories that detailed any medications the children were on and what was needed in the way of routine monitoring.

'This is William,' he said. 'He was born with a heart defect and had a cardiac arrest during

surgery as a baby which left him with mild cerebral palsy and epilepsy. And this is Simon, nine
years old, who's also a newbie this year and is a
type A haemophiliac.'

The photo showed a boy with dark spiky hair,
a delicate elfin face and a happy smile.

'Simon's here with his dad,' Mike continued,
'who also happens to be a new member of our
medical team. We're very lucky to have an emergency medicine consultant who has a special interest in paediatrics. Eli, stand up for a sec, will
you? Let's give you a proper welcome this time.'

Maya turned with everybody else but the
movement was no more than a reflex because the
chill that was rushing through her entire body
was freezing her ability to even think, let alone
direct her body to move. She certainly wasn't
making the slightest effort to contribute to the
welcoming hand clapping.

Eli...

It hadn't been simply a physical similarity that
had conjured up the ghost from her past.

It really *was* Eli.

And he had a *son*?

A nine-year-old?

Her brain might be frozen but it could still do
some maths. Eli had walked out on her ten years
ago. Straight into the arms of another woman
who'd become instantly pregnant?

Or was this kid closer to turning ten and discovering he was already a father had been the real catalyst, rather than the accident and its aftermath?

How ironic would that be?

The second round of applause faded and everyone was turning back to the front of the room as Mike carried on with the thumbnail medical histories of this year's campers, but for a long moment Maya still couldn't move.

Because as people turned and settled again she found she had a clear line of sight to the back corner of this group of people. To where Eli Peters was still standing.

Staring back at *her*...

He looked just as shocked as she was feeling.

As if this was the last thing he had expected. Or wanted. He almost looked...good grief... *angry*?

That snapped something back into place for Maya and she was back in control as instantly as she'd frozen. She was the one to break the eye contact and turn away. She probably looked as if she was completely focused again on Mike's presentation, but that couldn't be further from the truth.

She was being sucked back in time. Ambushed by a kaleidoscope of memories and emotions. Wounds that should have been long healed felt

as if they were being ripped open again and…
and it hurt.

More than she would have thought it possibly
could after all this time.

CHAPTER TWO

THE INTRODUCTORY TOUR of the medical facilities was more for the benefit of newcomers who needed to know basic things like where the defibrillators were kept, the rules for accessing controlled drugs and the protocols for emergency evacuations of any children who needed more intensive care than the clinic could provide.

'I'm going to give this session a miss,' she told Mike, having hung back as the group of people left the conference room after his briefing. 'I'd like to be there for the first boat coming in. I don't want to miss the chance to give Hazel her first hug of the year.'

Mike knew there was no real reason for Maya to tag along when she was just as familiar with the medical side of running this camp as the doctor and senior nurse who were going to help him lead the tour.

'Give her one from me, too,' he said. 'I'd come down to the jetty myself but I haven't seen the new ultrasound and X-ray equipment that got set up while I was in the States. I'll catch up with you soon.' Mike was smiling but there was a hint of a frown on his face at the same time. 'Are you okay, Maya? You're looking a bit pale.'

Maya managed a smile but it was an effort. 'I'm fine,' she assured him.

She couldn't tell him that she was still reeling from seeing the man that at one time she'd been so sure she was destined to spend the rest of her life with. Or that she was even more shocked that he had a child whose conception or birth might even overlap somehow with the time that she'd been living with Eli.

Trusting him.

Loving him with her whole heart and soul.

Staff were busy around them now. They were shifting tables and setting up photo boards and decorations. Like a mini conference, this would be where the camp attendees and their carers would come this afternoon to choose the activities they wanted to try and to talk about how they might need to be adapted to cater for any special needs.

As Mike left he pointed at a poster of a child with obvious cerebral palsy, dangling halfway down a cliff. The person in another harness right behind the child, helping him every step of the way, was Maya and they both had wide grins on their faces. Mike threw a grin of his own and a 'thumbs up' signal as he disappeared in the wake of the group, but this time Maya couldn't find one in response.

To her horror, she felt like she might even be close to tears and that was hardly going to reflect the joy that this camp promised to deliver. She knew she needed to get her head back together as soon as possible because she would be back here this afternoon to take charge of the area devoted to abseiling, rock climbing and the climbing wall which had custom holds and a system of harnesses that made it possible to give almost every child the experience of a vertical adventure.

Somehow, she had to face the explosion of memories that were threatening to overwhelm her and make a plan of how she was going to deal with this, and maybe the best first step she could take was to remind herself of why she was here.

The first boat carrying a group of the children and their carers from the main island could be seen approaching Reki Island as Maya arrived at the jetty. The local staff members, who had their own village on this private island, and jobs within the resort all year round, were gathering on the shore to greet the very different guests they would be helping to look after for the next ten days.

The women wore their uniform bright pink and white patterned dresses and the men had equally bright shirts and plain pink shorts. They all had colourful hibiscus or fragrant frangipani flowers tucked behind their ears and some had flower and shell necklaces draped over their arms, ready to be bestowed on the new arrivals as they came ashore.

One of the older women brought a yellow and white frangipani flower with a stem and went to tuck it behind Maya's right ear, but then she raised her eyebrows and grinned at her.

'Maybe it needs to be the left ear this time?' she asked. 'Did you get engaged or married since last year?'

'No…not this year, Moana.'

Oh, man… Could she blame the bright sunshine for how much she was having to blink?

Moana tutted. 'I don't understand why a gorgeous girl like you is still single.' She slipped a shell necklace around Maya's neck for good measure and gave her a hug. 'It's so good to see you.'

Maya let herself sink into the warmth and softness of the hug. Pacific women gave the best hugs ever. She felt better already, she decided as she moved to one side of the welcoming committee as they got ready. A couple of men were holding guitars and a few more had drums. Maya wasn't surprised to see a younger boy amongst them because, as always, there were plenty of children running around. What did surprise her was that this child wasn't Fijian. And that she recognised the delicate features of his face and the spiky hair over big dark eyes.

This was Simon.

Eli's son.

He was with Tevita, who was Ana's younger brother. Ana wasn't far away, watching them rather than the boat coming closer to shore so Maya knew she must have been tasked with looking after Simon. He looked…happy, she thought. He also had a shell necklace on and a flower behind his ear and his smile suggested he was very excited to be a part of the singing and dancing that would start as the boat tied up at the jetty. He qualified as one of the campers while he was here, because of his medical condition of haemophilia, but being on this side of the equation right now made him special.

Not that it was going to his head. Maya saw him look up at the bigger boys he was standing with and could see the way he took in a deep breath, proud to be one of them.

He looked like an adorable child.

He also looked very like his father.

It was Maya's turn to pull in a deep breath. She closed her eyes for a moment as well, willing herself to put the past back where it belonged, but it was harder than she expected. Because it was still hurting.

How could she not remember that first time she'd met Eli, when it had been so dramatic, both professionally and personally? She'd gone into the emergency department of a New Zealand hospital as part of a frontline ambulance crew to find the new English locum in the trauma response team ready to take over the management of a critically injured patient.

Maya had been riding the stretcher because she couldn't afford to take the pressure off an arterial bleed caused by a penetrating abdominal wound. The team had worked around her, stabilising the man's airway, breathing and IV access for fluid replacement before rushing him to Theatre so Maya had a central stage position to watch the most gorgeous man she'd ever seen at work. He'd noticed her, too. And he'd been the first person to notice, as they'd walked back to the ED after helping to get their patient to the surgeons, that some of the blood on her arm was coming from a deep scratch she hadn't realised she'd received.

'What have you done to yourself?'

'I have no idea. I did have to crawl under the car wreckage to get a line into him. I must have

got a bit too close to some mangled metal before the firies could cut him loose.'

Maya had liked how hard-core it made her sound. Or rather, she liked how impressed Eli had looked.

'It might need stitches. Let me look properly.'

It wasn't that serious. Maya was pretty sure this cut didn't need more than a spot of skin glue and a dressing at most and she was up-to-date with her tetanus booster, but Eli had held her arm gently in one hand as they rode the lift back to the ground floor and by the time he'd examined the wound they both knew it had begun.

And it felt like it could be the love story of the century.

They'd moved in with each other within three months. They were making plans for the rest of their lives.

As if they were providing a track for the movie of her life, Maya heard the joyous singing start around her—the strumming of guitars, the wonderful harmonies of voices and the heartbeat of the drums keeping the rhythm. It was the sound of the islands. A sound that Maya loved so much it was enough to make her smile through any pain her memories were trying to rekindle.

She'd been too young to know that flames that burned that brightly couldn't last. That even the glow of the embers could be completely snuffed out. They'd gone full circle, hadn't they? It had all ended just as dramatically as it had begun. With her being injured in the course of doing the job she was so passionate about, only this time it wasn't something that could be fixed with a bit of skin glue.

No... This was not the time or place to be thinking about *that...*

Maya snapped her eyes open, deliberately widening her smile as she saw the first passengers coming off the ferry Someone in a wheelchair being pushed by their carer was first and then a young girl came around them, almost running on prosthetic lower legs and feet, holding out arms that ended in points rather than hands.

'Maya... I'm *here*...' She raised her voice to be heard over the background singing.

'Hazel...' Maya didn't need to put any effort into smiling now. Even better, any unhappiness her brain had been trying to wrap around her was obliterated the instant she had this child in her arms. 'I'm *so* glad you're here, sweetheart. We're going to have *such* fun.'

But not quite yet, it seemed. Someone was running towards the jetty from where they'd parked an electric golf cart.

'Maya? Can you come, please? You're needed up at the helicopter pad.'

* * *

The call that led to the dispatch of Reki Island's helicopter to Nadi Airport had come in while Eli was touring the clinic, infirmary and minor procedures theatre that were all part of the island's impressive medical facilities.

'One of our first-time campers had what sounds like a syncopal episode after getting off a ten-hour flight from San Francisco. Fourteen-year-old who got a heart transplant three years ago and is travelling alone. The staff member meeting him got him to the first aid room and says he's got a rapid heart rate and seems a bit short of breath, but he's more distressed at the thought of missing camp than how he's feeling. It's a quick trip by chopper so I said I'd send one of our doctors to make the call about whether he needs to go to hospital and get checked out. Our pilot's standing by. I'd go myself but I can't abandon this introductory tour. Are you happy to go?'

'Of course.' Eli was already following Mike out of the clinic buildings. 'I'll need a life pack so I can get a twelve-lead ECG and monitor vital signs like his pulse oxygen level.'

'We've got a full resus kit, including a defibrillator, on board, just in case. And our paramedic is an experienced helicopter rescue crew member. She's going to meet you at the helipad. Her name's Maya. Come on, I can introduce you.'

Eli opened his mouth to confess how well he actually knew Maya but no words emerged. It wasn't as if it was going to make any difference to his ability to work with these children so there was no real reason for Mike to know that he might have decided not to come to Reki Island if he'd known Maya would be here. Or maybe he was processing the fact that she *had* ended up working on helicopters.

Of course she had.

The echo of his own voice from so many years ago felt like a reprimand. A familiar guilt trip that he'd been the cause of the wheels beginning to fall off the most significant romantic relationship of his life.

'You want to work on a helicopter crew? Are you kidding? Don't you think your job is dangerous enough already?'

'It's my dream job, Eli...this is what I do... it's who I am... You can get killed crossing the street, you know—why are you so paranoid about things that might never happen?'

'You know why...'

He could almost feel an echo of Maya's reassuring touch on his arm as well.

'Lightning never strikes twice in the same place, Eli. Nothing bad is going to happen...'

Except it had, hadn't it?

And maybe Eli was only beginning to realise how bad it had really been because he'd thought it was so far in the past it was completely buried. Until that moment in the conference room when he'd made eye contact with Maya for the first time in ten years and he'd felt a kick in his gut that was so powerful it felt like his heart had stopped beating for long enough to be alarming.

It was a punch of sensation that was a tangle of emotions he had no desire to try and untangle, but Eli could recognise the pain of loss, the struggle to get past something overwhelmingly huge and…and, *dammit*…there was also a unmistakable twinge of what he'd felt the very first time he'd laid eyes on Maya Thompson.

Unforgettable, irresistible, bone-deep sexual attraction.

How was he going to cope with that happening repeatedly for the next ten days? Or had that gut-wrenching reaction only happened because seeing Maya again had been so unexpected?

Unwanted…?

He was about to find out. A bright red electric vehicle was approaching the helipad behind the medical wing of the resort. Even from this distance he could see the wild dark brown curls of Maya's hair. He'd already felt the effect of making eye contact with her and that had been across a huge room crowded with other people. How much more powerful was it going to be when they were within touching distance of each other?

It had been like that from the first moment they'd met. An actual physical pull that had been like nothing Eli had ever felt before.

Or since.

Eli pulled in a deep, deep breath.

There was a professional reason they were about to be breathing the same air. He just needed to focus on that.

It was good that there was no time for anything but the briefest of introductions from Mike.

'Eli, this is Maya—a brilliant paramedic who can cope with anything. Maya, this is Eli—HoD of one of the largest emergency departments in London, with a special interest in paediatrics.' He grinned at them as the rotors on the helicopter were gaining speed. 'You guys are the A team for Reki Island's medical crew, that's for sure.'

She had to look at him as she nodded acknowledgment of the introduction. It was the briefest graze of eye contact but it was enough to notice that ten years had barely changed him. Maybe there were a few more crinkles at the corners of his eyes and deeper lines from his nose to that mouth, but those dark blue eyes were just as bright and there was no hint of grey in that thick brown hair that he always pushed back from his face if he needed time to think about anything.

Just like he pushed it back right then, as his polite smile faded almost instantly.

Maya's heart did an odd little flip at the familiarity of the gesture.

Or was it sinking like a stone because reading that gesture without having to translate it had suddenly opened the door to that private nonverbal language that was uniquely hers and Eli's? And she could feel the pull to walk closer to the door. To step through it, even?

How could she be that stupid?

She knew what lay beyond that door.

Heartbreak, that was what.

Her own equally polite smile also vanished and she reached for one of the helmets that the co-pilot, James, had ready for them as soon as the medical kits had been stowed. She jammed it on her head and climbed into her seat and hooked the straps of the safety belt over her shoulders and clicked the central locking system together. They were airborne within seconds.

'We've got a flight time of just under fifteen minutes,' Danny told them. 'The patient's in the first aid room and someone will be waiting to show you where that is. If necessary, we can transfer them to Nadi Hospital. Air traffic control will give us priority for landing and take-off.'

'Is it possible to get an update of whether there's been any change in the patient's condition, please?'

Oh, help... Maya had underestimated the effect of hearing Eli's voice through the inbuilt communication system in her helmet. It sounded as if he was close enough for his lips to be tickling her ears. How could it feel, after all this time, as if she'd heard that voice *that* close only yesterday?

'Sure thing.' Danny radioed through to the airport authorities.

'Do we have any history?' Maya's voice sounded oddly rough and she had to clear her throat. 'This is a first-time camper, isn't it? A heart transplant recipient?'

'I've got his notes.' Eli's voice was crisper now. Focused. He was looking down at his phone. 'Carlos Hermandez. Fourteen years old. Received a heart transplant two years ago due to heart failure caused by cardiomyopathy. Possibly hereditary—his father died suddenly four years ago at the age of thirty-five, leaving his mother with five kids to raise on her own. Carlos is the oldest. He's down to six-monthly checks by the transplant team and they've been delighted with his recovery. There's a note on his pre-camp check-up form to say he's an exceptional boy, responsible and independent. They can't see any problems with him coming to camp on his own and he deserves the privilege, given how much he does for his younger siblings.'

This was better. Maya was getting used to the sound of Eli's voice again. It helped that she had something else to focus on.

'And he had a syncopal episode?'

'At the luggage carousel. Apparently, he got too dizzy to stay standing. We don't know if he actually lost consciousness. The airport first aider reported a rapid heart rate and breathing and said he looked pale and sweaty.'

'Where did he fly in from?'

'Direct flight from San Francisco.'

Danny's voice broke into the conversation. 'Sounds like he's feeling better. Just scared he's going to have to go to hospital instead of camp.'

'Let's hope he doesn't,' Maya said. 'Have we got a list of his meds?'

'Yep.' Eli was scrolling the file he still had open. 'Immunosuppressant drugs, as you'd expect. An anti-hypertensive, lipid-lowering medication and…that's about it. No known allergies.'

Maya could see the shape of Fiji's main island coming into view. They would be landing soon.

'Fingers crossed it was nothing more than excitement causing a vagal reaction. Or nervousness, if he's never flown by himself before. Or maybe his anti-hypertensive has lowered his blood pressure a bit too effectively.'

'Could be an arrhythmia,' Eli said. 'The scar tissue from a transplant can create a pathway for re-entrant arrhythmias like atrial flutter.'

'We'd have to send him to hospital if there's any sign of infection,' Maya said. 'We can't afford to risk spreading something through a whole bunch of vulnerable kids.'

'No.' Eli's tone was sombre. 'Any sign of rejection is something else I'd be worried about. What happens if he's too unwell to come to camp?'

'The camp has insurance to cover an international medevac air ambulance service if it's necessary to send someone back to their own medical team. We've never had to use it in the five years we've been up and running, though.'

Maya could feel the surprise in Eli's gaze on her. 'Have you been involved all along?'

'Yes.' She didn't meet his gaze. 'I met Mike about nine years ago when he was on holiday in Australia. He'd just bought the island but he was full of the dream of using the success of the existing resort to set up the camp one day.'

The silence told her that Eli was reading way too much between the lines but she wasn't going to say anything else. She couldn't, when the thought occurred to her that she must have been with Mike around the time Simon had been born.

Anyway…for the sake of her pride as much as anything, Maya would much rather he thought she was—or had been—in a relationship than knowing she'd been left so broken when he'd walked away that it had always been an impossibility—with Mike, or anyone else for that matter.

Yes…let him think that she had got over him and moved on fast. That she had a life that wasn't going to be derailed by knowing he'd left her for someone else—and his baby.

An incoming international flight that had just landed was being held on the runway while the helicopter landed close to the terminal buildings. The empty arrivals hall made it easy to follow their guide as they carried their equipment and they were in the first aid room very quickly.

A tall, lanky teenager sat on the edge of a bed. His Spanish heritage was evident in his olive skin and mop of black curls. His distress at being kept in this medical facility was just as evident.

'Hey…' Eli put the backpack of medical gear he was carrying down on the floor, as if he knew it wasn't going to be needed in a hurry. 'Carlos? I'm Eli. Pleased to meet you.' He held out his hand in greeting and Carlos looked surprised but took his hand to shake it. 'I'm a doctor,' Eli told him. 'And this is Maya, who's a paramedic. We're both working at Camp Reki and we've been sent to see how you're doing. You had a bit of a dizzy spell, yes?'

Carlos shrugged. 'I guess... I'm fine now, though. You're not going to make me go to the hospital here, are you?' There was a plea in his dark eyes that told them it was the very last place he wanted to go.

'Not unless there's a very good reason to do so,' Eli said. 'How are you feeling now?'

'I'm good.'

'Can you tell me exactly what happened?'

'It was just hot in the baggage claim area and... I was looking around because I wasn't sure what to do and then I felt a bit sick and... I dunno...next thing I knew, I was on the floor and there were all these people staring at me.'

Maya had moved closer to put a life pack on the end of the bed. The machine beeped as she turned it on. She unzipped one of the pouches on the side and pulled out a blood pressure cuff. She smiled at Carlos.

'Can I check a couple of things while you're talking to Eli? Like your blood pressure and temperature—you know the drill, don't you?'

Carlos gave a resigned nod. Eli quizzed him

about how the flight had gone and how he'd been feeling in the last couple of days and had a quick look at his hands and ankles to see if they were puffy.

'Have you been having any joint pains?'

'No.'

'Any chills or feeling shivery?'

'No. Bit hot here, but I knew it would be. It's a tropical island, isn't it? It's supposed to be hot. I can't wait to go swimming. And diving around the reef.'

Maya was working quietly beside him. She clipped a pulse oximeter onto one of his fingers, swiftly wrapped the cuff around his upper arm and held his other wrist to take his pulse while the cuff inflated. She pricked his finger to get a drop of blood to test his glucose levels, and then pointed a thermometer at his forehead by the time the cuff was finishing deflating and figures were settling on the screen of the life pack.

'Temperature's thirty-six point five,' she said. 'BP's one zero five on sixty, heart rate's ninety-six, resp rate's twenty and pulse ox is ninety-eight on room air.'

Oh, wow… Had Eli forgotten just how efficient and calm Maya was when she was doing her job?

'That's all good, isn't it?' Carlos still sounded anxious.

'It is,' Eli said.

He could see that Maya was unravelling the wires required to do an ECG and see whether there was anything of concern in the heart rhythm or function, but that blood pressure and oxygen level in the blood was reassuring.

'Maya's going to stick some dots on you for the ECG and I want to listen to your breathing.' Eli turned to open the pack but Maya handed him a stethoscope. 'Deep breath,' he instructed as he positioned the disc on various areas over the lungs. 'And another one... Okay...lie back now and Maya can put the extra dots on your chest for that ECG.'

Carlos pulled up his tee shirt as he lay back on the pillows. The long scar down the middle of the teenager's chest was still in the process of fading.

Eli could feel how lopsided his smile was, but it was impossible not to think of how he'd feel if Simon had undergone such a major surgery.

'That's a pretty impressive war wound,' he told Carlos quietly. 'You've won a big battle, haven't you?'

Carlos grinned back at him with the same kind of cheekiness that Simon would have. 'I'm tough,' he said.

'You are,' Maya agreed. 'Keep really still for

a moment, though. I need to print out a copy of just how well that heart of yours is behaving.'

She handed the printout to Eli. It felt as though both Maya and Carlos were holding their breath as he examined each section of the twelve-lead ECG. When he looked up, it was Maya's gaze he caught first and...he knew she was reading his thoughts.

Like she had almost always been able to do...

When she smiled, it was impossible not to smile back at her. A real smile this time, because this wasn't about them. It was about a boy who was desperately keen to have some fun that he really deserved to have. They would need to keep an eye on him for a day or two but there was nothing to suggest he needed to go to hospital.

They both turned to Carlos and Eli's smile widened. 'How would you like a private helicopter ride to get to camp?'

CHAPTER THREE

BY LATE AFTERNOON all the camp attendees had
arrived on the island and the registration process
was in full swing.

Camp uniforms with the sky-blue tee shirts
and baseball caps were distributed. They had a
logo of a bright yellow circle for the sun fram-
ing a palm tree, Camp Reki and the year printed
beneath. Best of all, the tee shirts were person-
alised by having the name of the child embroidered beneath the right shoulder with a small
smiley face beside it.

There were queues in the conference area for
the uniforms and welcome packs that had all
the information needed for the medical facilities available and how to contact staff members.
Children and their carers were also lining up to
peruse all the activities available and sign up
for what they most wanted to do on their first
day tomorrow.

Maya was standing beside the photo montage
of climbing activities with an electronic tablet in

her hands and a smile on her face as she entered the name of a young girl who wanted to try the 'wall with the pretty bumps on it'.

'It's called a climbing wall,' Maya told Aliesha. 'And it's great fun.'

Aliesha nodded, as if she already knew that. 'I'm going to make friendship bracelets too,' she told Maya. 'I could make you one, if you want?'

'That's very sweet of you,' Maya said. 'And I'm happy to be your friend, but I think you should keep your bracelet. You could make one for your mum, too, maybe?'

As Aliesha skipped away with her mother, Maya turned to see a boy who was staring at the photos on the board with such an expression of longing that it tugged at her heartstrings.

She knew who he was. She'd seen him earlier today, playing a drum amongst the island boys down at the jetty.

She'd also seen his face on the screen at the meeting this morning where the staff had been briefed on the range of medical conditions this year's campers represented.

'You're Simon, aren't you?' she asked. 'You come from London, don't you?'

'How did you know that?'

'I know heaps of stuff,' Maya said. 'I know that you're nine years old and that you're here with your dad.' She frowned. 'I don't know if you've got any brothers or sisters, though.'

Simon shook his head. 'It's just me and Dad.'

Maya blinked. 'What about your mum?' As soon as the words left her mouth she knew she'd stepped over a boundary, but Simon wasn't bothered.

'I've never had a mum,' he said. 'Do you know that my dad's a doctor?'

'I do.'

'And that the hospital here looks like a tropical island? It's got palm trees and turtles on the walls and the rooms look like the huts. There's even a big tank in the waiting room that's got fish in it that are all different colours.'

'I do know that.' Maya nodded. 'I've been here before and I help out in the clinic sometimes.'

'Dad's there now. He's on duty till bedtime so he's going to miss the bonfire and the barbecue.'

'I'm sure he'll be able to come and have some dinner with you if nobody needs him. And everybody has to be there for the s'mores. It's like a camp rule.'

'What's a s'mores?'

'It's an American thing,' Maya told him. 'Mike, who's in charge of the camp, says it's not a proper camp unless you have s'mores. They happen when the bonfire has burnt out until it's just hot coals and everyone can get close enough to toast marshmallows. You get a cracker and put a piece of chocolate on it and then the roasted marshmallow and then another cracker goes on top of that and it makes a delicious, crunchy and squishy sandwich.'

'S'mores.' Simon nodded. 'Got it. I'll tell Dad he has to come for that bit.'

'Do you want to know why they're called s'mores?'

Simon nodded again.

'It's because they're so delicious that when they were first invented at a Girl Scouts camp, everybody wanted "some more" and it got shortened to "s'more".'

'If I tell Dad that and that it's a camp rule, he'll have to come, won't he?'

'Unless someone needs him,' Maya agreed.

But she was aware of a wash of relief that she wouldn't see too much of Eli on this first evening at camp. Even with something professional to focus on, like they'd had in their time with Carlos this afternoon, being that close to Eli had had its moments—like hearing his voice inside her helmet and the way he'd smiled at her when they'd both known there was no reason not to let Carlos come to camp.

Oh, *man*…she'd felt that smile right down to her bones.

'Hey…' Maya needed to stop any echo of how

that smile had made her feel. 'I saw you playing the drums today. You're very good at it.'

Simon ducked his head but his smile was proud. 'It was Tevita who showed me how to do it. He's Ana's brother. Ana's looking after me while Dad's busy. She's gone to get my tee shirts for me.'

Oh…it was a smile that came with the ease of being well-used, but that didn't dilute any of its warmth.

It was a smile so like Eli's…

With an effort, Maya crushed that persistent line of thought. She noticed that Simon was staring at the photos again.

'Do you want to try one of the climbing activities?'

He shook his head sadly. 'I can't,' he said. 'I've got haemophilia A. Do you know what that is?'

Maya nodded. 'It means that your body doesn't make enough Factor VIII, which is a protein that makes the blood able to clot.'

Simon nodded. 'So I can't do stuff like climbing mountains because, even though I get infusions all the time, if I hit something sharp like a rock I could still get bad bleeding. I've got a port, too, so I have to be careful not to bump it.'

'I understand,' Maya said. 'And I wouldn't suggest going anywhere near the real cliffs until you knew what you were doing, but the climbing wall is very safe. See those bumps and ledges? No sharp edges anywhere like real rocks. You'd be wearing a helmet and gloves, knee and elbow pads and you're in a harness and on a rope so you can't fall. The harness should cover your port and protect it, but if it doesn't we can sort that out. You've got someone right behind you, too. Someone like me, who's had lots of practice keeping people safe.' She grinned at the way Simon's face was lighting up. 'It's my favourite thing to do, teaching people how to climb safely.'

'I really want to do it.' Simon's voice was just a whisper.

'I've got one space left tomorrow morning in the first session,' Maya said. 'Shall I put your name in there? You can check with your dad later and make sure it's okay.'

Simon was sucking in an excited breath as he nodded. 'What time does it start?'

'Half past ten. After breakfast and the first swim for the day. It's easy to find. There's a signpost where the tracks cross near the front doors to the clinic building, but if you get lost it's on the outside of this building—round the back. You can't miss it—it's a huge wall covered in a rainbow of lumps and bumps.'

Bonfire nights were special. There was one on the first night for everyone to meet each other and any new children were shy and wide-eyed at the excitement of it all, the smell of food being cooked, the sound of drums in the background and the flicker of real flames from the fire in the central pit and the torches on tall poles that outlined the large grass circle.

There would be another bonfire on their last night at camp and Maya knew how different that would be, with children who'd gained so much more confidence, made friends for life and were ready to put on a performance and show off the songs and dances they'd learned.

Mike Davis was in his happy place, mingling with the guests, both children and adults, many of whom were catching up with friends from previous camps. Maya saw Mike spend extra time with Carlos and, judging by the way the teenager was shaking his head and smiling, he was being reassured that the medical incident at the airport had not been repeated. He then took Carlos to where a group of boys had gathered to watch the fire being stoked. Mason was there. And William, on his crutches. Maya found her gaze drifting, wondering where Simon was and whether he would like to be part of the group. She spotted him with Hazel and some of the younger children. Ana and another local woman were teaching them a dance near where the music was happening.

Maya had been busy in the last hour, shut in the supply rooms, double-checking that every emergency pack was fully stocked, that oxygen cylinders were full, that bags of fluid had not gone past their expiry dates and that the drug kits had everything she might need if she was called to an accident. Adding ampoules of tranexamic acid, a medication used to help control severe haemorrhage in trauma patients, had made her think of Simon.

Thinking of Simon made her think of Eli.

And thinking of them both made one question only get louder.

What had happened to Simon's mother?

'Penny for them?'

Maya turned swiftly to find that Mike was beside her. He held out a glass of what looked like fresh juice.

'Thought you might like a mocktail.'

'Thank you.' Maya accepted the drink. 'I was thinking of going to join in the dancing over there but I suspect the kids won't want big people taking over.'

Mike followed her line of sight. 'Ah…that's where Simon got to. I told Eli I'd keep an eye on him. I also told him to bring his pager and come down to the circle, but he's determined to go through the detailed medical background of every kid in camp.'

'Ha…' The word was more like a huff of breath. 'That sounds like Eli. Overcautious.'

She could feel Mike's steady gaze on her. 'You know him?'

'It was a long time ago.'

Mike was silent for a long moment. 'When I met you, I got the feeling that you'd been burned enough to put you off even thinking about a long-term relationship.' He cleared his throat. 'Would Eli Peters have had anything to do with that?'

Maya was silent long enough for it to be the answer to the question and Mike's next words were quiet.

'You okay with him being here?'

'As I said, it was a long time ago. It's ancient history.'

'That doesn't answer the question.' But Mike's gaze was gentle. 'I'm sorry I didn't know. I could have at least given you a heads-up. I only met Eli a couple of months ago—at a paediatric conference in Paris. I gave a talk about the benefits of medically complex kids being able to do normal stuff like going to camp and it came up in conversation when I met Eli at a dinner. Seemed like a match made in heaven when I heard about Simon.' His glance was quizzical. 'Did you know about Simon?'

Maya shook her head. 'That was more of a

shock than seeing Eli again, I think. Do you know what happened to his mother?'

'What do you mean?'

'He told me he's never had a mum. That it's just him and his dad.'

Mike shrugged. 'I don't know anything about that. And what did you mean about being over-cautious?'

'Eli's not a risk-taker,' Maya said. 'Which is partly why he's such a good doctor. He had adrenaline junkie parents who got killed by an avalanche when they went cross-country skiing in Switzerland. He was only about fourteen and his sister was even younger. They got brought up by grandparents. When he ended up working in emergency medicine it just reinforced his opinion that so many accidents were due to reck-lessness and I suspect that made him even more cautious.'

Mike was shaking his head. 'You're another adrenaline junkie,' he said. 'And I can't imagine you letting anyone clip your wings with the job and sports you love so much. I get why it didn't work out.'

Maya made a sound that acknowledged how unlikely a couple they'd been.

But it had never felt like that.

Quite the opposite. Even when she had indeed felt like her wings were being clipped, she'd been so sure they could work things out. That nothing could blow them apart.

And Maya had believed that until she'd fallen down that cliff. Literally and emotionally.

At eleven o'clock the next morning Eli Peters looked up from reading the repeat ECG he'd done on Carlos after giving him another thorough check-up.

'Thanks for coming back in this morning. I know it meant missing your first activity session, but we needed to make sure you were over whatever it was that made you unwell yesterday. I'd hate to think we'd missed something but, as far as I can tell, you're in great shape.'

'It's okay. Someone's going to get me some flippers and a snorkel and they're going to take me out in the lagoon. Just me…' Carlos looked as if he'd grown an inch since yesterday. 'They're really nice people here, aren't they?'

Eli nodded, smiling. 'They are. This is my first time here, too, and I'm really impressed. Did you enjoy the bonfire last night?'

'Yeah…it was great.'

'I only got there towards the end—when everyone was making those sticky marshmallow things.'

'S'mores.' Carlos nodded. 'They always have them at summer camps.'

'So I heard. We don't have them in England, but I might have to learn how to make them. My boy, Simon, thought they were the best dessert ever invented. Now...' He grinned at Carlos. 'How 'bout you get out of here and have some fun?'

Eli could get out of here for a while now, too, and he was planning to have a wander and see where some of the various activities were happening. He had a rough idea from the tour he'd done yesterday but it was information that he would prefer to have in greater detail. The tracks might be well signposted, but if there was an emergency like an accident he'd want to be able to get to the exact location as fast as possible.

He'd end his walk down at the beach and maybe he could find Simon, who might still be collecting shells. Or had he said something about going fishing after his swim?

Eli glanced at the pile of patient notes on the edge of the desk in this consulting room that he still needed to put away after going through them all last night. Simon had been disappointed that he'd missed most of the first night celebrations but the effort of getting really familiar with the medical history of every child at camp had been valuable. He'd felt as if he already knew everyone who'd come to the clinic this morning for routine checks or the administration of their long-term medications, some of which were done by IV infusion. Knowing what normal was for these children who needed more intensive monitoring meant that he'd be more likely to notice any change that could be the first indication of a serious problem.

Or was he justifying something he'd done for more personal reasons? Like avoiding spending any more time than necessary in Maya's company? That was hardly a strategy that he could keep up for ten days, was it? At some point, they were going to have to talk to each other.

How good would it be, Eli thought, as he clipped on his pager and headed towards the reception area of the clinic, if he and Maya could actually agree to forgive and forget and put the past behind them? If they could leave this tropical paradise having recaptured something of the friendship they'd once had, even?

Eli stepped out of the medical wing and stood for a moment looking at the signpost at the intersection of tracks near the front door. One yellow arrow was pointing towards the beach. Straight ahead was a forest walk loop and the opposite direction to the beach led to the climbing wall he'd seen on his tour yesterday. He'd go there first, he decided, and see how long it took to get there from the clinic because it was exactly the kind of location that you could expect an accident to happen.

He arrived to see a lively session in action, with each of the rainbow-coloured tracks of hand and foot holds reaching from the ground to the roof—a good ten metres in height—being used. A solid steel structure went up the sides of the wall and across the top, anchoring at least a dozen ropes. Children and instructors were attached to the ropes, wearing harnesses that looked as though they'd been specially designed to cope with any disabilities a child might have. They were wearing helmets and elbow pads and there were mats on the ground. The safety measures being taken were more than impressive enough to satisfy Eli.

Until he saw who was almost at the top of the wall.

Simon...?

Eli could feel the blood draining from his face as his heart rate accelerated. Fear morphed into anger. Where the hell was Ana? How had this been allowed to happen? Someone was responsible for this and he was going to find out who it was. They shouldn't be allowed anywhere near vulnerable children again.

Frozen to the spot, he watched as the instructor hanging beside Simon coached him into stretching his leg to find a foothold as they began their descent. The instructors and some of the older children were controlling their own belay devices. Adults on the ground were controlling the release of the ropes keeping other children safe. They were also clipped onto new metal fastenings on the wall every time they moved far enough, but that didn't stop Eli's heart dropping like a stone as he saw Simon lose his grip and swing away from the wall.

He could hear Simon's laughter, as though swinging in mid-air far enough off the ground to potentially kill him if he fell was the best fun he'd ever had. The instructor reached out a hand and Simon caught it. He was drawn back to the wall and found a hand grip. As the instructor turned to point to the ledge he needed to get his feet onto, Eli could see the face beneath the helmet.

Maya...

Of course it was. How had that not occurred to him as soon as he'd realised someone was breaking rules around here and being unacceptably irresponsible?

By the time Maya and Simon reached the ground, Eli was absolutely furious. He kept it hidden as he watched helpers unclip Simon's ropes and help him out of his harness and the safety gear. Maya kept her harness on and coiled a rope to hang from one shoulder, clearly ready to help the next child who was waiting for a turn on the wall, but Eli was walking towards her as she gave Simon a high-five hand-slap.

'Good job, buddy. It wasn't that scary, was it?'

'It was so *cool*.' Simon was grinning from ear to ear. 'Can I try it on the real cliff next time?'

'We'll have to see about that,' Maya said.

'Yeah…' Eli's tone was dry. 'That might be a good idea.'

Simon's head swivelled. So did Maya's.

'Hi, Dad…' Simon's voice was as small as he suddenly seemed. Guilt was written all over his face.

Maya looked from Eli to Simon. 'When I asked you this morning if your dad was okay with you doing this, you said he was.'

Simon scuffed the ground with his foot. 'I just said it was all good.' The look he sent his father made it clear that he blamed Eli for spoiling his fun. 'It *was* all good,' he muttered. 'Maya said it was safe and…' he was scowling now '…and I wanted to do it. More than stupid fishing…'

'Okay…' Eli kept his tone calm but it was an effort. 'Do you know where Ana is?'

'No.'

'Can you find the way back to our *bure*?'

'No.'

'I can take him.' The volunteer who had been

helping Simon take off his elbow and knee pads looked up.

'Thanks. Could you please take him to the reception area in the clinic? Simon?'

'What…?'

'You can wait for me in the room with the big fish tank.' It was an instruction rather than a suggestion. 'I'll come and find you in a few minutes and we'll have a talk about what activities you can do after lunch. Or, in fact, whether you deserve to be doing any at all.'

Maya watched how Simon's shoulders slumped and his head hung down as he was led away. He'd been so happy only a minute ago. So proud of his achievement of getting to the top of the wall. She flicked a glance at Eli, preparing to turn away.

'He was perfectly safe,' she said.

'He knew perfectly well he wasn't allowed to be doing a high impact activity like climbing. I'm going to go and find out what Mike thinks about this. You had absolutely no right to give him permission.'

'I didn't.' Maya was indignant. 'I explained how much safer the wall was than being out on a real cliff, but I told him he needed to talk to you about it.'

'You are aware that Simon has severe hae-mophilia?'

'I checked his notes,' Maya said, her tone cool. She resented the suggestion that she wasn't doing her job properly. 'I noted that he has a port-a-cath in place and that he's on infusions three times a week to boost his clotting factors. Our helmets are the best available and I gave him a padded harness and joint protection pads. I've had children who are a lot more medically frag-ile than Simon climbing this wall.'

'I'm sure you have,' Eli snapped. He'd low-ered his voice so no one else could hear their exchange. 'But do you have any idea of how re-peated bumps and bleeds into joints in a child with haemophilia can lead to life-limiting arthri-tis and the need for major surgery? Or how little it takes to cause an internal micro-bleed that can go unnoticed until it suddenly becomes a serious issue? Do you, in fact, ever take into consider-ation the possible consequences of *your* actions?'

Maya stiffened. He still blamed her for what had happened so many years ago, didn't he?

And why wouldn't he?

She'd never stopped blaming herself.

Maya took a steadying breath and spoke qui-etly.

'Has it occurred to you that you can't stop people doing something they really want to do for ever?' She risked making eye contact. 'That it might be a better idea for children to learn how to problem solve and do things safely than to put themselves in real danger by having a go at something like climbing when no one's watching?'

But Eli was glaring at her and she had to look away.

'Nothing's changed, has it?' His voice might be quiet but it was raw. He sounded disgusted. Or disappointed? 'Except that it's not enough for you to be doing what you want to do and flirting with danger when you're working—now you're using your time off to encourage kids to be just as irresponsible with their own safety.'

Maya's self-control was slipping. Okay, maybe she had good reason to regret some of her choices in the past and Eli had equally good reason to hate her for how they'd affected him, but this was more than unfair. It was a direct attack and she had to stand up for herself.

'You're being a helicopter parent,' she replied in a low voice. 'And you're still trying to wrap people in cotton wool and stop them being who they are. Or who they *want* to be. But you're quite right...'

She turned her back on Eli and began to walk away. 'Nothing *has* changed.'

CHAPTER FOUR

THE NIGHTMARE WAS always the same.

But this was the first time Maya had experienced it in more than a year and it had never happened on the haven of Reki Island as she slept beneath her mosquito net, her windows open so that she could hear the distant sound of waves washing onto the coral reef.

It was the sound that was the worst part of this recurring dream—the cry of a newborn baby. Maya could hear it so clearly but she could never find it as she ran from room to room in a building that felt like a deserted hospital, with long, long corridors that had too many doors on each side. The nightmare ended, as it always did, when she opened a door to find there was no floor behind it. She could still hear the cries of the baby as she fell, tumbling down the cliff, knowing that when she hit the bottom it would be the end of everything.

She woke with a cry of her own and sat bolt upright in her bed, wrapping her arms around herself in the hope that it would hasten the return of reality. She knew there was no hope of getting back to sleep so she got up, made a soothing cup of herbal tea and went outside to sit on the tiny veranda of her *bure* with its view onto the beach and the moonlight-gilded lagoon.

It was no surprise that the nightmare had found her again here.

Because the baby she could never find was her own.

Hers…and Eli's.

The fall had happened when she was at work. They'd been sent to a track that wound through a pine forest, up in the hills surrounding the city, to a mountain biker who'd come to grief on a steep downward slope and needed the assistance of the ambulance service. Maya loved calls like this that took her somewhere different and presented unique challenges. The biker had a badly broken leg and backup was needed to help carry him out of the forest when they'd splinted the fracture and given him pain relief. Maya had gone to pick up the pack she'd carried in. She'd stepped off the track without thinking, forgetting how slippery a thick layer of dry pine needles could be on a steep slope. It wouldn't have mattered because they should have cushioned her fall, but who could have known that beyond the screen of the trees to one side lay an enormous drop into what had once been a quarry?

Maya had been lucky to survive. A helicopter crew was called in to rescue her and she was transported to the emergency department where Eli was on duty. He wasn't allowed to treat her—only to hold her hand as she was assessed and stabilised. He'd been holding it tightly when the surgeon came in to give them the results of the CT scan that had added a significant injury to her spleen to the list of bumps and bruises and a few cracked ribs.

'We need to take you to Theatre to fix that laceration before you lose any more blood,' he'd told Maya. 'You're going to be fine but… I'm so sorry…you've lost your baby…'

Maya closed her eyes tightly as she remembered it, as if that might help her not to see the look on Eli's face as he'd heard those words. She felt herself curling her fingers into a fist at the same time—as if that could help her not feel the echo of the way his hold on her hand had loosened.

She could hear her own whisper. The words she hadn't really believed herself.

'It was an accident, Eli…it wasn't my fault…'

Simon wasn't smiling.

He wouldn't even look up at Eli as they went

into the treatment room at the medical centre the next morning.

'Hop up on the bed here, Si,' Eli said. 'Do you want anaesthetic cream on this time?'

'No. I don't need it.'

'Okay…' Eli put a mask on the pillow of the bed and then moved to the bench area. 'I'll be ready in just a minute.'

He prepared his tray as Simon climbed onto the bed, took his camp tee shirt off and put his mask on.

They might be in a new place today but this routine had been a part of their lives long enough for it to become as commonplace as getting dressed in the mornings. The regular infusion of a product that replaced the function of Factor VIII could prevent or reduce the frequency and severity of bleeding episodes in people with hae-mophilia A and it was a huge advance in treating the condition. Simon had had his port—a device that lay under the skin and connected to a vein—inserted when he was only twelve months old, which meant it was far less stressful to get IV access.

That didn't mean that care had to be taken, however. And Eli was always careful. He prepared a sterile tray with everything he needed, including the port needle, factor product and sterile syringes with saline and heparin. He could feel the silence behind him as he ripped open packets and dropped items without touching them.

A heavy silence. The kind you got when someone was far from happy. The talk he'd had with Simon last night about how he was only trying to keep him safe because he loved him so much had clearly not had the desired effect.

He mixed the factor product and filled the syringe. Then he carried his tray to put on the end of the bed that Simon was now sitting on.

'All set?'

'When can I start doing this by myself?'

'You already do some of it yourself. Like pushing the syringe plungers and putting pressure on afterwards so you don't get bleeding under your skin.'

'I want to do it *all* by myself. Other kids do.'

Ouch… Eli could feel the rejection.

'Other kids are older. They have their ports removed and they can inject themselves into a vein in their arm. The youngest person I know about who does that is thirteen years old.'

'I'm nearly ten,' Simon muttered. 'I could do it.'

Eli cleaned the skin over where the port was situated under his right collarbone. He anchored the device with two fingers of one hand and held the wings of the port needle with his other hand, ready to insert it. Simon didn't even flinch when the needle went through the skin.

He probably was just about ready to learn to inject himself. But Eli wasn't.

He attached the saline syringe. 'Want to pull back and make sure we're in?'

Simon's head was down. He wasn't even watching. 'Nah… I don't feel like it.'

Eli confirmed access, flushed the line and attached the factor syringe to inject the product slowly.

'So what's first on the agenda today? You're going kayaking, aren't you? And snorkelling? Or is it the boat trip out to see the giant turtles?'

Simon shrugged. 'I don't care. It's not what I really want to do.'

Eli let his breath out in a sigh. 'You know why the climbing wall isn't a good idea, Simon. There are so many other amazing things to do here. Why are you so determined to make not being able to do this one thing such a big deal?'

'Because…' Simon shrugged again and then his voice wobbled. 'Because it makes me happy…'

It was Eli's turn to be silent. He flushed the line again and then injected the heparin which would prevent the line clotting and causing a problem next time. He could hear Maya's voice in his head now, telling him he was being a helicopter parent. That he didn't let people be who they were, or wanted to be.

Had he always been like that?

He couldn't deny he'd worried about the risks that Maya faced in her work as a paramedic. He'd been the same with his younger sister, Sarah, when he'd become the protective older brother after the death of their parents. She'd been an adrenaline junkie, too, and that love of extreme sports had been responsible for her death, albeit indirectly. She hadn't been stupid enough to be skydiving herself, days after giving birth, but she couldn't stay away from her parachute club's exhibition of a group halo formation performance. Having parked on the roadside, she'd got out of the car to get the best view of her friends joining up in freefall, with Simon still tucked into his safety capsule in the back seat, and it was when she went to open the driver's door to head home that a speeding drunk driver had sideswiped the car and hit her, causing catastrophic injuries.

He could never forget that bolt of fear when he'd heard that news. It was automatic to clench a fist when he felt even an echo of it, as if it could prevent his fingers shaking the way they had when he'd scribbled that note to Maya in the midst of trying to find the quickest way he could to cross the world to be with his sister.

He'd written:

It's Sarah. It's bad. I'm sorry—I wanted to be here when you woke up but I have to go.
    I'll call you. I love you...
    Eli

It wasn't often these days that Eli felt a pang of the grief of losing Sarah but he felt it now, as he removed the needle from Simon's skin and pressed a wad of gauze onto the puncture site. It always came with the sadness of knowing that, in her induced coma, she wouldn't have been aware of how he'd sat beside her in the intensive care unit, day after day, with baby Simon in his arms. That she wouldn't have heard his promise that he would do everything in his power to keep her son safe. To make him happy.

He wasn't happy right now, though, was he?

'How 'bout we make a deal, Si?' Eli said quietly. 'You go on the activities you're signed up for today and I'll ask whether it's okay for you to do the climbing wall again tomorrow?'

Simon's head jerked up. 'Really? You'll let me do that?'

'You're growing up,' Eli said. 'You'll be able to take care of your own infusions before long and I know I'll be able to trust you to do it as carefully as when we do it together. I already trust you to be careful when you're at school or out with your friends. It shouldn't be any different just because we're at camp.'

'I knew you'd be mad at me,' Simon said with a grimace. 'But I thought the climbing wall was safe. Maya was looking after me.'

'I know, buddy.' Eli pulled off his gloves and ruffled Simon's hair. 'I wasn't angry with you. It just gave me a bit of a fright. Do we have a deal about today?'

'Yes...' Simon slid off the table. 'I've got to go and get ready. I can't wait to go and see those turtles.'

Eli watched him haul his tee shirt back on. He might not have been angry with Simon yesterday but he certainly had been with Maya. He'd blamed her entirely for what, if he was being really honest, was his problem.

He had been unreasonable.

He needed to apologise, didn't he?

The day had started badly for Maya, having not been able to get back to sleep after the nightmare and painful memories being stirred up.

It got worse that afternoon when her pager sounded, and she ran from the climbing wall session she was taking to arrive at the doors of the medical centre to find one of the resort's most popular workers looking very unwell as he was carried inside.

'Timi… What's happened?'

'He was sick,' one of the men told her. 'He said he had terrible pain in his chest.'

'Follow me.' Maya looked towards the reception desk. 'Who's on call?' she asked Moana.

'Dr Peters. We've paged him.'

'Okay… Tell him we're in the treatment room.'

Maya braced herself for the moment that Eli would come into the room. She had managed to avoid being anywhere near him since that unpleasant encounter at the climbing wall yesterday. She knew it was inevitable that it was going to be awkward having to work together, but by the time Eli came in, ten minutes later and rather out of breath, Maya was completely focused on her patient and, remarkably, it was easy to ignore any personal issues. She gave Eli a brief glance before turning back to the twelve-lead ECG trace that was emerging from the machine in front of her.

'This is Timi,' she told Eli. 'He's forty-six years old. He had sudden onset, ten out of ten, central chest pain radiating to his left arm and back that started about twenty minutes ago. He was diaphoretic, hypertensive and tachycardic when he came in and…' She walked towards Eli and for a long moment they both looked at the recording in her hands of the electrical activity in Timi's heart.

'Inferior STEMI,' Eli murmured. 'That's some impressive ST elevation in leads two, three and aVF.' He caught Maya's gaze. 'Do you have a Code STEMI protocol?'

'Yes.' A myocardial infarction that needed urgent intervention had a very clear pathway of treatment. 'I've already got IV access and he's had a bolus of five milligrams of morphine for the pain.' Maya stepped back towards Timi. 'How's the pain now?' she asked.

'Bit better,' Timi said.

'Score out of ten? It was ten out of ten when you arrived. What is it now?'

Timi closed his eyes. 'Maybe six?'

'We'll give you something more for that in a minute.' She took hold of his hand. 'It looks like you're having a heart attack, Timi. This is Dr Peters, who's going to look after you here, and then we're going to get you to hospital as quickly as we can so they can fix you up properly, okay?'

Timi was reluctant to let go of her hand. 'Will you come with me?'

'Yes. It's my job to go with people if they need to go to hospital. We've got a few things to do here first, though.' She turned back to Eli. 'Would you like me to activate Code STEMI and transmit this ECG to the hospital in Suva? I can get our pilot on standby as well. We'll need to transfer him by helicopter.'

'Has he had GTN and aspirin already?'

'Yes.'

Eli was looking at the oxygen saturation level and the blood pressure reading on the monitor. 'He's got a saturation of ninety-five percent on room air so we don't need any oxygen on, but we'll need to get a beta blocker infusion started to get that blood pressure under control. We'll need additional antiplatelet and anticoagulation therapy, too.' He picked up a stethoscope as he stepped towards the bed. 'Hi, Timi. I'm Eli. Can I listen to your chest, please?'

Timi nodded. He had his eyes tightly closed. Eli turned his head to speak to Maya. 'Let's top up that pain relief.'

Maya listened to Eli's questions as she flushed the IV line and administered the first of several medications Timi was going to need. It felt as if she'd stepped back in time to when it was normal to be working alongside Eli. Something to look forward to because, even though they maintained a perfectly professional distance at work, it felt as if it was knitting their lives closer together.

It didn't feel like that today.

Working with Eli might not be as awkward as Maya had feared but that professional distance was only a fraction of the personal distance between them. They might as well still be on opposite sides of the world.

Eli was finishing quizzing Timi on his medical history.

'Have you had any broken bones or major surgery in the last six months, Timi?'

'No.'

'Been to the doctor for anything recently?'

'No… I'm healthy. I've been off the smokes for a year now, Doc.'

'That's great.'

'I'm trying to lose a bit of weight, too. But it's not so easy when you've got a wife who's such a good cook…' Timi was smiling now as the pain relief began to kick in.

Eli was running through an extensive checklist of any contraindications for any of the standard medications for starting to dissolve the clots blocking Timi's coronary arteries when Mike arrived.

'I heard you called a code,' he said. 'The chopper will be ready to take off in a few minutes and I can go with Maya to help monitor Timi.'

Maya felt a wash of relief, knowing she wouldn't have a return trip with Eli when there wasn't a patient to focus on, which would only make that personal distance even more painfully obvious.

'What can I do to help now?' Mike asked Eli.

'We're going to need another IV line. Maya's already done a great job with the initial assessment and treatment but I'd like to get the fibrinolytic therapy underway ASAP.'

The praise was unexpected.

So was the look Eli gave Maya after Timi's stretcher was loaded onto the helicopter and Mike was already on board.

'See you later,' he said. 'Come and find me when you get back? Please?'

Maya nodded. 'Of course. You'll want to know how Timi's doing.'

She turned to get into the helicopter but felt Eli touch her arm and turned her head. He didn't need to say anything because she could still read his eyes. It *felt* as if she was reading his mind.

He wanted to talk to her about more than how Timi was doing. It looked as though he wanted to apologise.

And suddenly that personal distance seemed to have shrunk. Because Maya wanted to talk to him, too. She had an apology of her own that was long overdue.

The beaches of Reki Island were stunning at both sunrise and sunset, and when Maya met Eli by the jetty the light was just beginning to fade and the first hint of a pink blush was staining the sky.

'How's Timi?' Eli asked.

'Fine, thank goodness,' Maya responded. 'He went into VF en route and we had to defibrillate him but we got him back into sinus rhythm on the first shock.'

Eli whistled silently. 'I can imagine how tense the rest of the flight was.'

'We waited until he was out of the catheter lab. No neurological deficit. He's got two stents, one of which fixed a total blockage in the left anterior descending artery, and he was feeling very happy to still be alive.'

'I can imagine. He's a lucky man to get a second chance at life.' Eli looked up at the darkening hues of the sky and the reflection of the colour on the still waters of the lagoon. The beach was deserted. 'Fancy a walk?'

'Have you got time?'

Eli nodded. 'Mike's on duty at the medical centre. He'll only page me if there's a real emergency. And Simon's at movie night with his mates and what looked like an endless supply of popcorn. He couldn't be happier.'

For a long time, they walked in silence along the stretch of damp sand, close to the tiny waves uncurling beside them. When the sun had sunk low enough to make them need to shade their eyes as they looked up, they spoke at the same time.

Only two words.

'I'm sorry…'

There was another moment's silence. Maya wanted to say more. Too much, perhaps, because she couldn't find the words she needed to even begin. Eli broke the silence.

'I'm sorry about the way I spoke to you yesterday,' he said. 'I *am* overprotective of Simon. I have been ever since he was a baby and it only got worse when I discovered he had haemophilia.'

'How old was he when you found out?'

'He was in the accident that injured my sister Sarah so badly. The paediatrician who examined him thought the bruising was odd, given the protection of the car seat he was in. By the time I got there from New Zealand, they'd done the tests.'

Maya was frowning. 'Why was your baby in your sister's car?'

'Because Simon was Sarah's baby.' It was Eli's turn to frown now. 'He's not *my* baby. I'm his uncle.'

'But he calls you Dad.' Somewhere in her confusion was a wash of relief. He hadn't walked away from her to be with another woman. To be a father to his own baby.

'I adopted him to try and keep him safe legally, although I don't believe his biological father even knows of his existence.'

'You never told me that Sarah was pregnant.'

'I didn't know. I hadn't seen her, except in video calls, since I went to New Zealand and she'd gone off to go backpacking around Europe and there were always good reasons that she didn't call often. I guess she didn't want to tell me because she knew I'd be worried about her. Maybe she wanted to prove she could live her own life without her helicopter brother hovering over her.'

Maya bit her lip. She shouldn't have said that. It was perfectly understandable that Eli was overprotective. Simon had needed special care ever since he'd been handed to Eli as a tiny baby when his mother was too sick to care for him.

'I spent more than a week sitting in the intensive care unit by Sarah's bed,' Eli added. 'But she never woke up. I often had Simon in my arms. I felt like his dad from the moment they gave him to me. The first thing I did after they turned off the life support for Sarah was to go and pick him up and hold him. I told him that I was always going to look after him.'

'Oh, my God…' Maya could picture Eli sitting there, holding a baby as he was grieving the loss of the baby sister he'd been protecting ever since their parents died. She could feel the prickle of tears at the back of her eyes. 'I'm so sorry, Eli. I...didn't know.'

It felt like no excuse at all. She hadn't been there when the man she'd loved so much was going through something so awful. And then it struck her.

'That was why you left New Zealand in such a rush. And why you never came back? Why didn't you *tell* me?'

'You'd just been taken to Theatre—after that awful row we'd had about you still working even though you were pregnant—and suddenly I was trying to get through to the hospital in London to find out what was going on and trying to book flights that would get me there as soon as possible. I barely had time to get home and grab my passport and pack a bag.' He shook his head. 'But I did tell you. I left you a note. I said something bad had happened to Sarah.'

She remembered. She'd read that note a thousand times.

'You said you'd call,' Maya said quietly.

'I did call.' Eli's voice was expressionless. 'Whenever I could, which wasn't that often, I admit, because I was trying to learn how to care for a baby and spend as much time as I could with my sister, and then I had to organise a funeral and try and make plans for the future. I left voice mails. I texted. Until I couldn't even do that because all I got was some automated network voice telling me that the number was not in service.'

'Of course it wasn't. It had been lost somewhere on that cliff I fell down. The battery would have died. Why didn't you call the hospital?' Maya hadn't forgotten what it had been like to come round from the anaesthetic to find that Eli wasn't there. To wait and wait for a visit that never happened. The pain, both physical and emotional, had been horrible. The grief—and guilt—she was feeling about the loss of their baby only made it a hundred times worse.

'I did,' Eli said. 'But you'd been discharged by then. I got hold of a friend in ED and he found out that you'd gone up north to stay with your family while you recuperated. He said he could try and get the number but...' Eli pushed his fingers through his hair. 'There was too much I had to deal with and...and I was still shocked about you losing the baby. About that fight we'd had. It felt like a mess I didn't have the energy to deal with right then. When I hadn't heard from you by the time I needed to resign from my locum position remotely and arrange to have personal stuff shipped back to the UK, I guess... I don't know... I was hurt. Angry. I felt kind of powerless. My life had been completely derailed.'

Maya understood all of that.

Maya remembered feeling exactly like that herself. Arriving home after more than a month away, recovering from the accident and surgery, doing well but still nowhere near a hundred per-cent, to find any trace of Eli had been removed from the apartment they'd shared. The life she'd thought she would have for ever had been sim-ply erased.

'I had to focus on what really mattered,' Eli said. 'And that wasn't how I was feeling. It was Simon.' He blew out a long breath. 'You didn't try and call *me*...'

'No.' Maya stopped walking. She stared at the final, bright halo of the sun sinking swiftly below the horizon, sucking the colour from the sky as it disappeared. 'I...' she cleared her throat '... I didn't think you'd want to hear from me. I knew it was my fault...'

'The accident?'

'No. Well, yes...but that *was* an accident. I'm sorry about the baby. I'm sorry I didn't listen to you when you said I needed to step back from working on the road. I thought it was far too early to worry. Maybe I needed more time to just get used to the idea—it wasn't as if we'd planned on having a baby. I'm sorry, Eli...' The tears Maya had been holding back were finally es-caping. Hot, slow, painful tears. 'I'm sorry about everything. About the baby and Sarah and not calling you…'

'I'm sorry, too. For everything that happened all those years ago. And for taking it out on you when I found that Simon had managed to sneak into a climbing session. He…um…wants to come again tomorrow, if that's all right with you?'

Maya looked up, startled. 'You're okay with that?'

'It's what he wants,' Eli said. 'And I know, from personal experience, that it's not a good idea to stop someone trying to be who they are. It can end in tears.'

Maya swiped at the tears on her cheeks but she found a hint of a smile. 'That's true. I'd be happy to see him back. I'll take good care of him.'

'Thanks.' Eli looked around them. 'It's getting dark. Mike's probably wondering where you are.'

Maya's eyebrows rose. 'Why would he be? Oh…' She was remembering something else now—being okay with letting Eli think that she was in a relationship. Being less than completely honest with this man had led to a decade of guilt and self-recrimination and it simply wasn't acceptable to let history repeat itself.

'Mike and I are just friends,' she admitted as she began walking to the nearest track leading away from the beach. 'I've never…' Her voice trailed into silence. What could she say? That she'd never found another relationship? That she'd never found anyone that could have taken Eli's place? That she'd never found the courage to trust anyone that much again?

Eli was close behind her, otherwise she might not have heard his soft words.

'Neither have I…'

CHAPTER FIVE

MAYA DIDN'T HAVE any bad dreams that night, but she didn't sleep particularly well either.

Why hadn't she tried to call Eli all those years ago?

She could—and had—excused herself by the fact that she had been badly hurt, both physically and emotionally, but even during the worst period of her life she'd been aware that she was being selfish. She'd made it all about her. *Her* surgery, *her* miscarriage, *her* being abandoned by her boyfriend...

She hadn't even tried to find out what had happened to Eli's sister.

She'd pushed aside the fact that Eli was the other parent of the baby that had been lost.

She'd simply refused to tap into the heartache of knowing that Eli was probably feeling just as hurt and confused and sad as she was.

Instead, she'd endlessly replayed snatches of the awful interaction that had been the last time they'd spoken before he'd vanished from her life.

They'd had to wait for an operating theatre to become available. Her physical discomfort had been under control but the silence in that private room as Eli stared out of the window was full of a level of pain that the medication couldn't touch.

'This...this is why I hate you doing such a dangerous job. You could have died, Maya. Our baby did die...'

'You're blaming me? It was an accident, Eli. Accidents happen.'

'It didn't need to. You knew you were pregnant but you decided it was way too early to worry about it. You decided to take the risk— even when I said it wasn't just your safety you were risking. You didn't really care, though, did you?'

'Are you saying I don't care that I lost the baby?'

'I'm saying you don't care about the risks you take. And that makes me wonder how much you care about anything. Yourself. Our future. Me...?'

Maya had turned her face into her pillow.

'Go away, Eli. I really don't need this right now.'

It was a new shock to discover why Eli hadn't contacted her and it reignited that awareness of how badly she had treated him. He had been going through more than the pain of a physical injury and the loss of an unplanned and very early pregnancy. He'd had to cope with the stress of getting back to the other side of the world as quickly as possible and then the loss of his sister. On top of that, he'd had the overwhelming responsibility of a tiny, vulnerable human put into his hands at the same time. And he'd done it without her support. She'd told him to go away and he'd done so wondering how much she really cared about him. She wouldn't have blamed him for hating her enough to not try and contact her at all.

But he had. Again and again. He must have assumed, as she had, that her phone was still clipped to her belt in the bag of patient property along with all her other clothing. He must have decided that she didn't want to talk to him. That she really *didn't* care that much.

Had it changed anything for him to learn that she hadn't received any of the text messages or voice mails?

As much as learning what Eli had had to deal with had changed things for Maya?

They both needed time to process that intense conversation they'd had last night, but when Maya walked into the dining room a short time later she saw Eli and Simon at the buffet table, choosing their breakfast food. She picked up a bowl and headed for the fresh fruit salad that was always her choice to start the day and as she turned she found Eli watching her.

And smiling.

'Hi, Maya.' Simon was beaming at her. 'Dad says I can come and do the climbing wall again this morning if it's okay with you.'

'It's more than okay,' Maya told him. 'I think it's a brilliant idea.'

She smiled back. At both of them.

Unexpectedly, it felt as if it might be a good thing that her path had crossed with Eli's again like this. As if it might be possible to find forgiveness—on both sides—and make peace with the past. To heal enough to be able to rekindle some kind of friendship?

More than friendship…?

Maya sucked in a shocked breath. What was she thinking?

It had been bad enough recognising that connection was still there between them—the one that had created a whole nonverbal language. Did she need to remind herself again that getting her heart broken once had been more than enough?

Of course she didn't. So why on earth was she having to push away something that felt like… longing?

Maya reached for some coconut milk yoghurt to spoon onto her fruit, giving an imperceptible shake of her head to complete the process of dismissing that line of thought.

Feeling at peace when it came to Eli Peters was all that she needed to find. That would be life-changing enough in itself.

Eli knew that Maya was expecting Simon at the climbing wall session but the way her face lit up when he arrived suggested that she was genuinely delighted that he was being allowed to do it again.

Clearly, she hadn't expected Eli to come as well. He saw a flash of wariness in her eyes that was disturbing. Did she think he had come along in order to watch her every move in case she made a mistake and Simon got hurt? That he was here to rain on Simon's parade the way he probably had on hers when they'd been together, despite—or perhaps *because* of—being so much in love with her, when he'd criticised her choice of a career and her even riskier preferences for hobbies and exercise?

He raised his hands in Maya's direction, palms up, in both greeting and a gesture of submission. 'I'm just here to watch,' he said. 'Simon wants me to see what he can do.'

'I have to go and get my helmet and harness on now, Dad. And my elbow and knee pads. I'll be back soon. Don't go away, will you?'

'Not going anywhere, buddy. Do you want some help with the safety gear?'

'We've got plenty of helpers who know what they're doing,' Maya said.

Were her words mild encouragement to step back and let Simon be more independent? If so, it was fair enough. Eli gave a single nod.

During the long hours of a broken night, Eli had been sucked back into the past and, with the benefit of hindsight, he could see that, to Maya, it would have felt like he was holding her back from living her best life. He couldn't blame her for accusing him of being overprotective with Simon either. But, in his defence, he hadn't realised it at the time. Maybe it had been woven into every breath he'd taken, thanks to the trauma of losing his parents and being too young to take on the frightening responsibility of keeping his little sister safe.

Simon was already heading towards the equipment area but he turned back. 'Can I try the blue route today, Maya? Or the green one?'

'You did the orange one last time, didn't you?'

'Yes…and you said I smashed it.'

'You did.' Maya was grinning again. 'How 'bout we go up one level and do the red route today? Maybe the blue one next time.'

'Okay…' Simon ran off happily to get ready.

'What colour is the easiest?' Eli asked.

'Yellow. You can see that there are handles to hang onto and steps for easy foot positions. They're the routes that we use for the more disabled kids and there's an option to go sideways and not get to any real height. We can actually use it for children in wheelchairs. Or who need to be on oxygen.'

Eli could see a little girl skipping towards them. 'And for kids like Hazel?' He shook his head, more than a little surprised that a child with no hands or feet would have climbing down as a choice for camp activities. But he was smiling as well. 'How amazing is her attitude to life?' he added quietly.

'She's an inspiration all right,' Maya agreed. 'But I don't think she did Yellow more than once. She gives climbing the same determination she does everything else in her life. I wouldn't be surprised if she conquers Black eventually.' She held her arms out for an enthusiastic hug and then sent Hazel off. 'Simon's over there,' she told her. 'I think he likes climbing as much as you do.'

Eli was looking up at the wall. 'Who's doing the black route at the moment? It looks like Carlos.'

Maya nodded. 'Turns out he's been climbing for a year or so at his local gym. He's wanting to practise his abseiling so he can come on the real cliffs later this week.'

'Who's that doing Red?' Eli shaded his eyes. 'Oh…it's Alice. I've seen her at the medical centre a few times. She comes in to do her respiratory exercises with the physiotherapists.' He could feel himself frowning. 'She's frail, isn't she? Looks like just a bump would break her arms or legs.'

'She's been struggling with her cystic fibrosis for the last couple of years. We almost didn't accept her for camp this time but her family said she was desperate to come and they're afraid it might be her last chance.'

Eli could remember scanning her notes. 'She's on the waiting list for lung transplant, isn't she?'

'Not yet. She put it off for as long as possible. She's recently had the work up tests and counselling but she would have had to stay within a certain distance of the hospital in case donor lungs became available and that would have meant she couldn't come to camp. She made a deal with her family that if she was allowed to come here she'll go on the list as soon as she gets home. That's her older brother, Jake, who's on the wall beside her. He's come as her carer. He's nineteen and planning to go to medical school.'

'That doesn't surprise me. Growing up with

siblings who need complex medical care is often the catalyst for a career choice.'

Her sideways glance at him was almost shy— as if Maya wasn't sure if she should broach a more personal subject? 'Like it was for you after your parents died?'

Eli shrugged. 'They were killed instantly in that avalanche so that should have encouraged me to become a paramedic or search and rescue expert.' He offered Maya a wry smile. 'Guess I knew I would prefer a nicely controlled indoor environment for my work. If anything, my choice was influenced by Sarah's penchant for ending up in Emergency when she'd fallen over rollerblading or got thrown off the naughty pony our grandparents bought for her.'

But it was food for thought. Had he chosen his specialty knowing that he might be able to prevent other families going through the grief of losing someone who hadn't been careful enough? To save someone like Sarah who couldn't resist the adrenaline rush of fun that had an edge of danger?

Maybe, one day—if they could ever get that close again—he could tell Maya how his relationship with his own sibling might have contributed to breaking what he and Maya had found together.

'You don't need to worry about the ponies we

have here if Simon's going on one of the forest or beach treks. They're all totally bombproof.'

'I thought they would be. I think he's got that on his programme for tomorrow.' But Eli was clearly thinking about something else as he stared up at Alice. 'Is she okay?'

Jake had his arm around Alice, who seemed to be hanging in her harness, making no attempt to move her hands or feet to new holds.

But Maya was no longer beside him. Climbing the wall like a spider, she had reached Alice's level within seconds. They were only about halfway up the wall but, to Eli, it still seemed a long way to be off the ground without a safety harness and rope.

It was impressive. It also reminded Eli very strongly of that single-minded focus on someone in trouble that had first attracted him to Maya Thompson and he could feel a much stronger flash of that attraction that had been so disconcerting when he'd first seen her again on the island. This time, his body responded in a way he hadn't felt in years.

About ten years, to be precise...

So long, he'd forgotten how powerful it was to feel every cell in his body coming alive like this.

Her confidence was just as sexy now as it had been then and Eli could see, with the benefit of being older and wiser, that it wasn't that she was throwing herself into something without thinking it through. The intense expression on her face advertised her lightning-fast assessment of every move she was making. When she stopped, she had her feet on two different holds that protruded from the wall, was hanging onto a higher lump with one hand and, with the other, he could see her taking Alice's pulse as she was talking to Jake. On top of planning her own movements on her way up, she had probably been thinking about how to approach her assessment of Alice, hadn't she?

Wow...

Had he forgotten just what an impressive person Maya was?

How proud he had been of her?

He hadn't forgotten any of it, of course. He'd just buried it to protect himself from the pain attached to all those memories. It should have been easier than it was to bury it again now as he watched Maya helping both Jake and Alice down to ground level as swiftly as possible.

'Alice had a bit of a dizzy spell,' Maya told Eli. 'And some muscle cramps.'

Eli could hear the wheezing sounds of her breathing that suggested a level of airway obstruction that needed attention.

'Let's get you to the medical centre,' he said. Jake was looking very worried. 'She seemed okay when we did her breathing exercises this morning. She did say she had a bit of a headache but she still wanted to do the climbing. I should have realised something wasn't right...'

Eli's heart went out to the teenager. He could remember all too easily what it was like to feel this protective of a younger sister. As if sometimes the weight of the whole world was resting on your shoulders.

'You're doing an amazing job of looking after Alice,' he told Jake. 'This isn't your fault, okay?'

'Have you got your inhaler with you, sweetheart?' Maya asked.

'I've got it.' Jake pulled the device from his pocket. He was clearly practised in helping Alice use it and doing something to help was the best way to distract him from blaming himself.

'We'll get the harness and all the pads off you, too.' Maya was already undoing fastenings. 'Being overheated won't be helping. Have you had plenty to drink in the last couple of days?'

Alice nodded, too focused on her breathing to say anything.

'I've been trying to make sure she's getting plenty of fluids,' Jake said. 'I know that people with CF are at a much greater risk of dehydration because they lose so much more salt in their sweat. But maybe I miscalculated how much she needs. It's hotter here than at home and Alice is doing more physical stuff, isn't she?'

'The symptoms could be caused by dehydration,' Eli agreed. 'But we need to rule out any kind of infection.' He crouched and held his arms out to Alice. 'Best way to get you inside quickly is for me to carry you. Are you okay with that?'

Standing beside Alice, Maya caught the full force of the smile that Eli was giving the young girl as he reached out to lift her into his arms. It was genuine and caring and irresistible because it was so warm. She could *feel* it, all the way down to her toes.

She knew what it would feel like for Alice to be swept up and held like that, too. It might have only been in fun, when Eli sometimes picked her up and carried her into their bedroom but she knew exactly how strong those arms were.

How safe they could make you feel.

The sigh she could hear beside her seemed to echo exactly what she was thinking as she watched Eli carry Alice around the corner of the building, heading for the medical centre. She looked down to see the disappointment on Simon's face.

'Dad's not going to see me climbing, is he?'

'Maybe not this time,' Maya said. 'He needs to help Alice. She's not feeling very well.'

Simon's nod was resigned. 'He likes looking after sick kids.'

'He's very good at it,' Maya said. 'He's good at looking after anybody,' she added. 'Kids or grown-ups. People who are sick or have had accidents and hurt themselves, sometimes very badly. And you know what the best thing about him is?'

'What?' Simon was scuffing the ground with his foot.

'He really cares about the people he looks after.'

Maya had known that about Eli from the first time she'd seen him at work and she'd never seen that level of care slip. He'd always been particularly good with kids and that was one of the things she loved most about him.

Had loved, she corrected herself instantly, but the damage had been done.

Had she really just reminded herself of how much she'd loved this man?

Or felt a pang of yearning for something more than friendship to be rekindled?

Bad idea...

Because it was confirming a fear she'd held at bay for the last ten years. A fear that she had never really got past that breakup. That she never would. And if she had been too afraid to go into another serious relationship ever since, surely it was a no-brainer not to get any closer to the man who'd done the damage in the first place?

The man who'd left her waiting…

Hoping against hope for something that was never going to happen?

Maya knew exactly how disappointed Simon was feeling. She put her arm around his shoulders. 'He said to say sorry. And he told me to stay here and make sure you had fun.'

She had offered to go to the medical centre and help with Alice's care, but Eli had already picked Alice up and she knew that Mike would be there to assist and they could call in any other staff they needed, like physiotherapists to help try and clear Alice's lungs.

The glance Eli had given her as he declined her offer and told her to stay and help Simon with his climbing session had said a lot more. She knew he was trusting her to look after his son and, no matter that the echoes of the past were making themselves felt, she wasn't about to let either of them down.

'Tell you what,' she said. 'Why don't I give my phone to my friend Josefa, who helped you get your safety gear on, and ask him to take some photos and videos of you climbing and then we can show your dad later?'

'Oh…can we?' The glow was back on Simon's face. 'That's a *great* idea, Maya.'

Maya took Simon to the dining room after the climbing wall session but let him sit at a table with other kids, including his friends Hazel, Carlos, Alice and Mason, to eat. There was a rest period after lunch when Ana took him back to his bure because Eli was still busy at the medical centre, but when she went to the beach to help with the sand sculpture competition that afternoon, he turned up a short time later.

She handed Eli her phone to let him catch up on Simon's achievements on the climbing wall that morning. Being on a section of the beach that was shaded by palm trees made it easier for him to see the videos and photos.

He was impressed.

Simon was as proud as punch.

So was Maya.

'Look at that,' she said. 'The way he's feeling for the holds and making sure he's secure before he shifts any of his body weight. And there… that's called a bump. He's a natural.'

Oh…she'd had to lean rather close to Eli to point to the small screen. She could smell his aftershave. Except that this smell was *so* familiar and he'd never used aftershave that she knew of. This scent was simply Eli.

And it gave her a sudden curl of sensation deep inside her body that was more than a little disconcerting, especially when it came with an awareness that she was only wearing a bikini beneath the sarong tied in a knot over her shoulder and tucked in at her waist because she was planning to have a swim when the sand castle competition was finished.

Thank goodness Simon broke the moment and pushed closer to try and see what they were talking about.

'What's a bump?' he asked.

'It's where you get a hand hold but you can tell it's not really going to work so you reach for another one straight away.' Maya nodded at him. 'Look... I'll start it again. You're good at this stuff, Si.'

His dad was also nodding. 'I'm proud of you,' he said. 'Maybe we can find a place for you to keep doing this when we get back home.'

Simon's grin couldn't have been wider and Maya caught her breath. She felt oddly proud of herself now as well. She'd been the person who had introduced Simon to this activity and contributed to the pleasure—and confidence— he'd gained from it. And if she hadn't stepped in his father might have banned the sport as being too dangerous and he wouldn't have this record of his efforts this morning, which would be a memory he could treasure and show off to his friends at home.

She tapped the screen of her phone. 'Put your number in,' she said to Eli. 'I'll forward the album.'

The thought occurred to her that she would have Eli's number then and they could keep in touch, but she pushed it aside. Why would either of them want to do that?

'Are you going to help with our sandcastle?' Simon asked his father.

'Sure.' But Eli raised an eyebrow as he looked down at the odd shape on the damp sand they were standing on. 'It's a castle…?'

'Sand sculptures can be anything,' Maya said. 'Simon's decided to make an octopus.'

'And adults are allowed to help?'

'Yes. It's kind of a family thing because some campers need more help than others. There are staff members to help the kids that are here without family or carers. Or they gang up together, like Carlos and Hazel over there. Looks like they're making a boat. Are you sure you don't want to join them, Si?'

'Not now that Dad's here.' Simon was still smiling. 'But you can still help, too, Maya, if you want to.'

Eli caught Maya's gaze as he handed back her

phone. 'That would be great,' he said softly. 'If you don't have other stuff you have to do.'

'Not at all.' The invitation was giving Maya a wash of something warm. A feeling of being welcome? Wanted, even? Whatever it was, she liked it. A lot. 'I'd love to help.'

For the next hour, they carried buckets of water to keep the sand damp, collected a lot of shells and some sticks to use as tools and then sculpted a head for the octopus and long, tapering legs radiating outwards. The overall effect was that of a rather misshapen starburst.

Simon stood back to look at their creation. 'He's a bit wonky.'

'He's fabulous,' Maya declared. 'And see these cockle shells we found?' She held up a round white shell. 'If you stick those on his legs, upside down, they'll look just like tentacles.'

Simon pushed a shell into a sand leg. 'Hey… you're right. But we'll need an awful lot of them.'

'We'd better get on with finding them, then. I think we've only got another half an hour and then the judges will be coming to look at everybody's sculptures.'

Eli watched Simon race off with his bucket to find more cockle shells and then he smiled at Maya.

'You're good with kids,' he said. 'Have you got any of your own?'

She avoided looking at him as she shook her head, reaching for another shell to push into the sand of the closest leg. 'Never felt ready, I guess.'

There was a beat of silence.

'Because of the miscarriage?' Eli's voice was soft. 'I'm sorry, Maya. I...should have tried harder to reach you. I was so caught up in my own life going belly-up that I didn't think enough of how hard things were for you. And—'

'It's okay,' Maya interrupted. She didn't want to be reminded of how many reasons he'd had to feel angry with her. 'Let's not keep apologising. We were both young. We made mistakes.' She looked up to catch his gaze. 'It would be nice if we could put it behind us.'

Eli held her gaze. 'It would,' he agreed. And then he smiled. 'We're both older and wiser now. I can recommend having a kid. It felt like a bomb had gone off in my life to start with, but I wouldn't be without Si now. He makes every-thing...worthwhile. Special. It might only be the two of us but it...feels like family.'

Maya simply nodded and smiled back. She couldn't say anything else because Simon was already on his way back, his bucket brimming with the common shells.

'I found these big, long curly ones, too,' he

said, holding out one of his treasures. 'How cool would they be for his eyes? Like kind of laser beams or something.'

'Exactly like laser beams.' Eli admired the shells. 'You're a genius, Spider-Man.'

Maya sat very still for a minute, watching as Eli and Simon threw themselves into decorating the octopus, crawling around on their knees, their dark heads close together as they positioned the eye shells.

They were a family, these two, and she could feel just how special their bond was. She'd been honest when she'd told Eli that she'd never felt ready to have children. Maybe she hadn't even given it much thought, what with focusing on her career and her sports. She got her fix of being with kids every year when she came to this camp, too. But being here, like this—as part of the Peters' octopus creation team—had changed something. Maybe it was because of what Eli had said about Simon making his life worthwhile. Or, more likely, it was due to feeling like she was part of the family after being included in that bond, even for a short time.

This was something important that was missing from her life.

Maybe she *was* finally ready to move on. To find a new relationship and have a child. To have a family—and a bond like that—of her own.

CHAPTER SIX

THE NEXT DAY dawned as blue and sunny as the last and the sea breeze that ruffled the hibiscus and frangipani flowers on the bushes near every bure was as warm as always, but the camp staff members, gathered for their daily briefing before breakfast, were talking about a weather system brewing in the South Pacific Ocean that was threatening to turn nasty.

'It's being closely monitored by the Fiji Meteorological Service,' Mike told them. 'It was noted as a low-pressure area northeast of the Solomon Islands last week but it's been upgraded to an off-season tropical cyclone this morning and has been named Lily. Currently, Vanuatu is on high alert and preparing for the cyclone to arrive in around seventy-two hours, but it's not expected to affect any Fijian islands—even those of us closest to Vanuatu. We might get some wind and rain and bigger waves but I'll keep you posted on any warnings.'

Eli walked out of the meeting area with Maya.

'Have you been here on the island in bad weather before?'

She shook her head. 'I think Mike's a bit more worried than he's letting on. Not that we couldn't keep the kids entertained if we got shut indoors for a day or two. It's more the problems it could bring if we needed to evacuate someone for emergency treatment. Bad weather would ground the helicopter. Even transport by boat could be cut.' She was frowning now. 'How's Alice this morning, do you know?'

'I'm just about to find out. She'll be in the medical centre for her respiratory physio about now and I'm heading over to give Simon his factor infusion.'

'Do you think her symptoms yesterday were due to just dehydration?'

'She certainly responded to some fluids. It would explain why her oxygen levels and forced expiratory volume had dropped noticeably. Dehydration thickens the mucus and makes it difficult to clear the lungs. We gave her bronchodilators, anti-inflammatories, antibiotics. She was feeling—and looking—a lot better by the time I got to the beach to help with the octopus.'

Eli threw a quick grin in Maya's direction. 'I know it was for the kids but I haven't had that much fun in quite a while.'

'It *was* fun,' Maya agreed. 'Simon was so

happy with his prize for the most artistic sculpture.'

'He was. But I think he was even happier when he was invited to sit in the sand boat with Carlos and the other kids when the tide was coming in. I got some great photos while you were swimming.'

'Show me?'

He opened the images on his phone and watched her smile as she scrolled through them. It made him smile, watching *her*.

He'd been watching her yesterday afternoon, too. Brief glances at first as they'd worked together helping Simon build the octopus, but after the judging she'd announced that it was time for a swim and had untied the sarong she was wearing to reveal her bikini.

Eli had been unable to politely avert his gaze. Maya's body didn't seem to have changed at all, despite the years that had passed. He knew every inch of that gorgeous, tanned skin that was suddenly on display. He knew what every curve felt like. *Tasted* like… He'd never found anyone else that turned a sexual encounter into so much more. He'd had sex since being with Maya—of course he had. But he'd never truly made love, had he?

And until that moment he hadn't realised how much he'd missed it.

At least Maya didn't seem to guess what he'd been thinking when she dropped her sarong into the basket where she had her phone and pager safe from the sand and looked up, straight at him. She'd simply asked him to give her a wave if he heard her pager go off.

She handed him back his phone. 'Brilliant photos,' she said. 'Can I keep this one to go in the Camp Reki newsletter?'

Eli looked at the row of children in the boat, laughing as they continued the game of leaning over the sides to scoop handfuls of seawater to throw at each other.

'Yes, of course,' he said.

He took another glance at the photo as Maya tapped in her phone number and forwarded the photo. All the kids, including Simon, had such incredibly happy faces that it brought a lump to Eli's throat. Simon was going to remember this camp for ever.

So was he. For more than the good times he was sharing with his son. He would never think about this camp without remembering reconnecting with Maya. Hopefully, they were undoing some of the emotional damage they'd both been living with for the past decade so those memories wouldn't be tinged with regret.

He had her number in his phone now. He

could easily add it to his contacts, but did he want to do that?

To stay in touch?

Yes…if it was possible to retrieve some kind of friendship from the fragments of what they'd once had together, how could he resist?

'You'll get some more great photos this afternoon.' Maya was turning to head down another track. 'The pony trek in the forest is very photogenic. I hope Alice is well enough to do it. She's horse mad—just like I was at her age.'

Like Sarah had been, too.

Eli found himself thinking about his sister as he headed for his morning clinic in the medical centre. Remembering being Jake's age and living with that fear that he might lose the person he was trying so hard to protect because they were the sunshine for *his* world. He'd stepped back as they got older and began to go their own ways. Sarah had been desperate to go travelling and he'd taken the opportunity to have an adventure of his own. He'd gone to work in New Zealand, where he'd met Maya. Had part of the attraction been that she had that adrenaline junkie gene like Sarah? Like his parents?

His protective instincts had become divided as he'd fallen more and more in love with Maya. In those first, terrible days watching over Sarah in the intensive care unit, Eli had wondered if it would have made a difference if he'd stayed more focused. If he'd kept watch over her more carefully instead of being persuaded that she was more than capable of looking after herself.

She had promised to keep herself safe. She'd said—like Maya had—that what she chose to do for her work or hobbies wasn't really any more dangerous than anything else in life. How ironic was it that she *should* have been totally safe when she'd only been watching the skydiving?

However unjustified it had been, that hadn't stopped a small part of Eli's grief—anger, even—being directed at Sarah because she'd been so passionate about a high-risk sport. And laid at Maya's feet for not only feeling the same way about taking risks in life but having distracted him from what had been so important when he'd been Jake's age—watching over his little sister. If he hadn't been in New Zealand, he could have been with her that day. He would have been, if he'd just become an uncle and wanted to make sure that both Sarah and her baby were being looked after. She might have been uninjured if she'd been opening the passenger door of the car instead of stepping out onto the road.

Eli pushed the overly-familiar thought away. 'What ifs' never helped.

Like the one that had resurfaced so strongly after talking to Maya. What if he'd tried harder to get hold of her?

But he couldn't, could he? Not when he was in the middle of experiencing what he could be setting himself up for in years to come by being with Maya—a repeat of this agony of losing someone he loved this much.

It had seemed so much wiser to let it go. And so much easier because he had a tiny baby who needed his full attention.

The serious young man was with his sister in the treatment room of the medical centre when Eli arrived. Jake was watching Alice as she did her positive expiratory pressure exercises.

'Breathe in through your PEP,' he encouraged her. 'Now blow out. Harder…bit harder…keep the blue bobble between the lines… That's better… Okay, one more time…'

'How's it going?' Eli asked.

'Peak flow's down on yesterday,' Jake told him. 'We're doing some extra physio to see how much Alice can clear her lungs.' He picked up a small plastic cylinder. 'You ready to huff now?'

Alice nodded, not speaking to save her breath. She took the cylinder and closed her lips around it. Jake held a strip of tissue in front of her. Alice took in a slow, deep breath, held it for a few seconds and then breathed out as hard as she could, making the tissue flutter. She bent her arm to cough into her elbow.

A short time later, Alice tested the strength of an expelled breath again, blowing as hard as she could into the peak flow meter.

'Better than it was,' Jake said, but he didn't sound happy.

'Any more headaches?' Eli asked.

Alice shook her head.

'Dizziness?' The query elicited another head shake. 'Temperature?'

'Normal,' Jake said.

'Not feeling sick?'

'No.' Alice was biting her bottom lip. 'I'm okay to do stuff today, aren't I, Dr Peters? I really want to do the pony riding this afternoon.'

'Let me have a listen to your chest,' Eli said. He was frowning as he put the earpieces in place, remembering something else from Alice's notes. 'Aren't you allergic to horses?'

'It's only a mild allergy.' Alice was scowling at him. 'I'm fine if I take some antihistamines.'

Eli caught Jake's glance and he could understand all too well that note of helplessness he could detect. There was good reason to stop Alice going on the pony trek, but they would be stopping her doing what she desperately wanted to do and…it was possible that this was going to be her last camp. Her last opportunity to do something that brought her so much joy.

'Our camp paramedic will be there,' he reassured Jake. 'She's got a kit that can cover any airway issues. I'll be there, too. My son Simon is really looking forward to it.'

Maya loved the pony treks and always put her name down to assist. She loved the reminder of her teenage years with grooming and putting the tack on ponies of all different sizes. There were special saddles, including one that was almost a chair for children like Eliana who had been born with severe spina bifida and had a passion for all animals, but especially turtles and ponies.

There were extra staff and volunteers involved, with up to three people for each child and pony—one to lead it and another on each side to help any children who had issues with balance or hanging on, like Hazel or William with his cerebral palsy, but there was never a shortage of helpers. There was a particular magic in vulnerable children interacting with large, gentle animals that was always a highlight of an already rewarding camp experience for adults and children alike.

Amongst about fifteen children in the group, Simon was riding a brown pony called Toffee. Ana was holding the lead rope but Simon

had said, very firmly, that he didn't need people walking on either side. Behind him, Jake
was leading Alice on a shaggy grey pony called
Smoke. Having been asked to keep a close eye
on Alice, Maya was walking not far behind her.
She had a pack on her back that was heavier than
usual because she'd added a small oxygen tank
to the usual range of trauma gear like dressings,
splints and bandages.

Eli fell back far enough to walk beside Maya
along the wide track that had been carefully
woven through the forest. It was deliciously cool
in the shade of enormous trees like kauri and
mahogany and so green with a mid-level layer
of palm trees and ferns covering the ground.
The pop of colour from wild orchids was pretty
and the sound of children's laughter and excited
squeaks was just as musical and joyous as any
birdsong it was drowning out.

When Maya looked sideways, she caught the
expression on Eli's face.

'Gorgeous, isn't it?'

'Unbelievably so.'

'It's my happy place,' Maya said. 'Well, the
whole island is—especially when it's full of
kids.'

The smile they shared gave that happiness a
dimension that Maya had almost forgotten ex-
isted. She knew that sharing an experience with

someone you knew made it special because it somehow made it more real when it was going to become a shared memory. But sharing an experience with a soul mate—which was what Eli had once been for her—took it to a whole new level. It forged bonds. Or reinforced them.

Could it be capable of mending them, too?

Would she want that?

That flash of longing she'd had when she'd seen Eli for the first time after they had talked on the beach that night was there again, squeezing her heart, but Maya didn't get a chance to even think about it before it evaporated. The pony trek was coming to an end and it was when Jake lifted Alice from Smoke's back that they could hear her breathing. A wheeze that was audible from too far away.

But Alice was smiling as she threw her arms around her pony. 'Take a…photo, Jake… I want to…remember today…' She pressed her cheek against Smoke's neck. 'That was…so…cool.'

Being unable to speak more than a few words before trying to grab another breath had both Eli and Maya walking towards Alice.

'Have you got a nebuliser mask and salbutamol in your kit?'

'Yes. And oxygen.'

Alice gave Smoke another kiss before he was led away but then she seemed relieved to sink to the ground. She leaned forward, clearly in respiratory distress. Jake had gone pale.

'If you kneel behind Alice, you can support her to sit up and lean forward,' Eli told him. 'That will help make breathing easier. We're going to set up a nebuliser mask to give her some bronchodilator medication. Did she take the antihistamines and use her inhalers before coming on the trek?'

'Yes. I made sure she took everything.'

Maya filled the chamber of the nebuliser mask with medication and attached it to the oxygen cylinder.

'I'm just going to put this over your face, Alice,' she warned. 'It should help make your breathing a bit easier.'

'Is it her CF?' Jake asked. 'Or is it asthma from her allergy?'

'Doesn't matter right now,' Eli said quietly. 'We need to treat the symptoms, not the cause.' He'd unrolled the IV kit from Maya's pack and tightened a tourniquet around Alice's arm. 'I'm going to pop a needle into your vein,' he told her.

'I shouldn't have let her come on the trek,' Jake muttered. 'I knew it was risky.'

Alice pulled the mask off her face. 'I don't… care…' she said, with difficulty. 'Best…day… ever…' She held the mask to her face again and Maya pulled the elastic band back into position.

Ponies and other children were being taken away and someone arrived in a golf cart. 'Do you need to get Alice back to the medical centre?' they asked.

'In a sec.' Eli nodded. 'Sharp scratch, Alice...' He slipped the cannula into a vein and removed the needle seconds later.

Maya handed him tape and then a clear plastic covering to secure the IV access.

'Thanks.' By the time he'd flushed the line, she had removed any air bubbles from the tubing attached to a bag of saline and it was ready to provide fluids and keep the line open.

This time, Eli thanked her with no more than a graze of eye contact but it was as clear as him having spoken aloud and it took Maya straight back to times they'd worked together in an emergency in the past. Back to the first time he'd ever made eye contact with her, in fact—when she'd known that the world as she knew it had just tilted on its axis.

Right now, it felt as if nothing had ever come between them.

They travelled together with Alice on one electric vehicle, with Jake following in another. There was no improvement in Alice's breathing by the time they arrived at the medical centre. Mike came to assist Eli and they started a continuous salbutamol infusion and began administering other medications including adrenaline. Maya put electrodes on Alice and monitored her vital signs at regular intervals. Her heart was beating too fast, her attempts to breathe were too rapid and shallow and the oxygen levels in her blood were too low.

An hour later, there was still no improvement and it was obvious that Alice was becoming drowsy. And confused.

'Where's… Smoke?' she asked. 'Did I…fall off?'

'No, sweetheart.' Maya squeezed her hand. 'You didn't fall off. You're a great rider. You did the whole trek without even looking like falling off.'

Alice's eyes were drifting shut but she was smiling. Her lips were starting to look a little blue as the level of oxygen in her blood decreased further.

'She sounds a bit better,' Jake said. 'I can't hear her wheezing now.'

Eli took him further away from Alice and Maya knew he was explaining that not hearing the wheezing was not a good thing in this case. It meant that Alice was getting too tired to keep struggling to breathe and was in danger of a respiratory arrest, which would necessitate intubation and mechanical ventilation. She needed to be in an intensive care unit as quickly as possible.

Maya stayed with Jake as he made contact with his parents, ready to answer questions or take over the call if he became too emotional to speak. Her heart was breaking for this big brother who was trying so hard to hold things together when he was clearly terrified that he might be put in a position to make decisions that were too huge to do alone. He had tears rolling down his face by the end of that call.

The only decision that had been made in the wake of the shocking news was that Alice and Jake's parents were going to head to the airport immediately and wanted to be called again in an hour when they got there to see what flights might be available. If possible, they wanted to speak with Alice's doctor at that point.

By then, Mike and Eli had Alice intubated and ventilated. The helicopter was waiting to transfer them to the biggest hospital available in Fiji, but they were already talking about having to medevac Alice to New Zealand which, at less than four hours flight time, was the closest country to get more expertise and advanced intensive care facilities. Eli and Maya would accompany Jake and Alice and stay until the next decisions were made. Mike and the other medical staff on the island would work extra shifts and cover everything needed on the island. Ana would be with Simon at all times to care for him.

As they settled Alice onto the helicopter's stretcher and arranged all the equipment they needed to ventilate, monitor and keep on top of the medications their patient required, they could hear Mike talking to her parents.

Jake caught Maya's gaze as she was checking the IV lines on Alice's arm that were connected to the bags of fluids. 'What is he talking about?'

'ECMO,' she told him. 'It stands for Extra Corporeal Membrane Oxygenation.'

'It's a machine that can take someone's blood and oxygenate it and put it back in their body,' Eli added. 'It would be an option if Alice was getting worse despite mechanical ventilation and intensive care but it's not available here. That would mean taking her to New Zealand or Australia.'

Jake looked horrified. 'She wouldn't want that.' His voice broke. 'She told me she didn't even want a lung transplant. She was only going to go through it because it was what Mum and Dad wanted.'

Maya knew that it was emotion that was making Eli's eyes so dark. She could almost feel his touch herself when he reached out to grip Jake's shoulder.

'It might not come to that, mate. Let's just take this one step at a time, okay?'

'You're coming with me, yeah?'

'Yes. We'll be with you the whole time.'

They were with Jake as Alice was cared for in the ICU in Suva as each hour passed and her condition didn't improve. They were there when his parents found flights that could get them to Fiji by late the next day. And they were there when Alice's body finally gave up because it wasn't getting enough oxygen and she went into cardiac arrest and died despite the best efforts of everyone involved, including Eli and Maya.

They sat with Jake as they waited for his parents to arrive and it was the most heartbreaking experience in Maya's life. Alice's big brother was absolutely devastated. He was also afraid that his parents might blame him for allowing her to do the pony trek that had caused the allergic reaction that had been enough to tip Alice into a downward spiral that couldn't be reversed.

'Tell them,' Maya said softly. 'Tell them what Alice said to you.'

Jake had his head in his hands. 'What? That she thought she'd fallen off Smoke?'

'No.' Maya put her arm around Jake's shoulders but her gaze was holding Eli's. They both had tears falling. 'That it was her best day ever...'

* * *

It was late by the time they arrived back on Reki Island the next day. Mike told Eli that Simon was already asleep and that Ana was in the bure with him.

They went into the medical centre and talked Mike through everything that had been done for Alice. That her parents had, of course, been devastated not to have been with their daughter but they could take comfort in knowing that Jake had always been her favourite person in the world and she would have known he was there with her. They'd sent a message for Mike to thank him for giving Alice such a magical time at camp over the years. They were going to send him a copy of the last photograph taken of Alice—when she had her arms around her pony's neck and the happiest smile imaginable on her face. They would be holding that image in their hearts, they said, for the rest of their lives.

There were tears. Comforting words and hugs. And then Eli walked with Maya as she finally headed to her own *bure*, one of the closest to the beach. They could hear the whisper of waves breaking and the rustle of the wind in the leaves of the palm trees.

They got to the steps that led up to her small veranda, but Eli didn't turn away to go to his own *bure*. He could see Maya's face so clearly in the moonlight and how could he leave when he could see just as clearly that she was utterly exhausted and so deeply saddened by what had happened?

But he didn't know quite what to say to try and comfort her either.

In the end, he simply opened his arms and held her when she instantly stepped into them. He kept holding her until he could feel the tension in her body start to subside, breathing in the scent of her hair as she softened in his arms.

And then she looked up at him and he could actually feel himself falling.

Back into a space he knew as intimately as his own body. A space that had—and *could*—only be there if Maya was sharing it.

It was *their* space. Where there was nothing to keep them apart—physically or emotionally. Where they could give, and receive, what had often felt like everything anyone could possibly need.

It felt as natural as taking his next breath to press his lips against her hair. Against her forehead as she raised her face. And then she tipped her head back even further and he thought it was so that she could look up at him, but she had her eyes closed and her lips parted—just a little— and he could *feel* that she wanted this as much as he did. So he kissed her lips.

Just softly. Briefly.

But he couldn't quite lift his head again and his lips hovered over hers, not quite touching but close enough to feel them. Or perhaps he was feeling the crackle of electricity between them, just for a heartbeat. And then another.

That infinitesimal gap was suddenly gone and this kiss wasn't going to be nearly as soft. Or brief.

This was a *real* kiss. A kiss that took Eli back, not only into that space that could only be there with Maya, but back in time, as though the last ten years had simply evaporated.

Except that he knew they hadn't.

That this kiss should not be happening.

So he broke it, trying to move far enough away this time to not feel any irresistibly magnetic pull.

Maya's whispered words jerked him to a halt. 'Don't go… Please…'

She needed him. He could hear it in her voice and see it in her eyes. He could feel it in his heart, or possibly in his soul.

And there was no way Eli was going anywhere.

CHAPTER SEVEN

THE NEWS ABOUT Alice spread like wildfire through the camp.

Maya could almost feel it happening as she walked on the beach as dawn was breaking the next morning. Shocked whispers as staff members and caregivers were informed. Gentle conversations with the children that were cushioned with cuddles and tears.

There were clouds on the horizon this morning but they only made the sunrise more dramatic. The sea breeze was strong enough that it should have made it a nuisance to have to keep pushing her hair out of her eyes, but Maya found it comforting. Because it reminded her of how Eli had brushed tears from her face last night and buried his fingers in her hair as he'd kissed her for the first time in ten, oh, so long years and yet it felt *exactly* the same.

Well…not exactly. They'd both gained a decade more experience of life, including the pain of their own failed relationship, and that had added a depth to this physical touch that could never have been there otherwise. This was so much more significant than it ever had been, too, because the comfort of intimate human touch, even in the wake of an overwhelmingly emotional experience, had to be based on trust. For Eli and Maya to trust each other this much had made that first kiss, and the slow, tender lovemaking that came later, something extraordinary.

Maya turned to face out to sea and closed her eyes as she took a deep, slow breath. The wind kept her hair off her face now. She could smell the salt of the sea in the air and hear the sound of waves crashing on the reef outside the lagoon. She still felt sad and emotionally drained after being so involved in the tragic loss of Alice yesterday, but surrounding those feelings—like a huge internal hug—was the comfort she had found in Eli's arms.

More than that even, because twinkling like small stars amongst it all was something that felt like astonishment.

How amazing was it that the love she had felt for Eli had apparently never died, even though it had been so deeply buried? That it was still there, like the tiny embers of a fire that could, if she wanted it to bc, quite possibly be reignited. That unique ability to communicate without words had made her think that Eli had been just as astonished, but nothing had been said aloud. Maya didn't want to say anything that could potentially break something so new and fragile. Or perhaps it was because she couldn't allow herself to even hope that this meant something when she knew how much it would hurt if Eli didn't feel the same way.

Or maybe the real problem was that he would feel *exactly* the same way. As they'd both said— or rather, fired as verbal weapons at each other— nothing had changed. Even if Eli did feel the same way as she did right now, getting too close might mean they were setting themselves up to be reminded of how incompatible they actually were. And that might hurt even more than this rekindled attraction turning out to be only one-sided.

The distraction of remembering every moment of last night, before Eli finally left her *bure* so that Simon wouldn't wake to find himself still under Ana's care, wasn't going to help Maya face a difficult day ahead. Or maybe it was, because she would be able to tap into the strength of knowing that, even if it was unwise, or Eli wouldn't—or *couldn't*—acknowledge it, he still loved her.

He had told her that with his body last night.

The sound of a helicopter getting ready to take

off made Maya turn. She hadn't realised that Eli's *bure* was so close to the nearest path down to the beach until she saw him on his balcony. He lifted a hand in greeting and by the time she walked closer to the fringe of palm trees he had come down onto the sand.

They both looked up as the helicopter flew overhead, still gaining height. Maya raised her hand to farewell Mike, whom she knew would be on board and possibly looking down at the beach. She touched her hand to her heart, too, hoping that he would take the gesture as a sign that she would be thinking of him today, while he was in Suva to assist Alice's family with arrangements for the sad journey they would be making to go home.

'Are you okay?' Eli asked.

Maya was about to give the automatic response that she was fine, but she could see something in Eli's face that made her change her mind.

'Those poor parents,' she said softly. 'They've lost something so precious. They'll be devastated.'

Even having lived with the knowledge that their daughter had a terminal illness couldn't lessen the grief for Alice's parents at losing one of their children.

But Eli knew that she was talking about something else as well. That she was opening the door to a discussion that neither of them had probably ever imagined they would have.

'At least they have each other,' Eli said just as quietly. 'I'm sorry I wasn't there for you, Maya.'

Eli and Maya had lost their baby. Being so early in the pregnancy hadn't seemed to lessen that impact enough. They'd never shared that grief and maybe that *had* made it harder for both of them. They'd lost their relationship as well. Grief upon grief.

'I'm sorry, too, Eli.'

'It's a long time ago.'

She nodded. 'But sometimes—for me—it feels like yesterday.'

Eli's half-smile was poignant. 'Me, too.'

He pulled her into a quick hug and then, with his hands on her shoulders, he bent his head and kissed her.

It was nothing like the kiss that had escalated into passion last night but it was slow. And so tender it broke Maya's heart.

'I'd better go,' Eli said as he broke the kiss. 'Simon should have got himself dressed and ready for breakfast by now.' He turned before she had time to say anything, striding off as if he needed to escape.

Maya didn't follow him immediately. It had been a huge subject to broach. A huge thing to acknowledge that they had both let each other down by not offering support. Maybe they both needed at least a bit of space.

She watched him walking back towards his *bure*. Catching movement from the corner of her eye made her glance up to see that Simon had come out on the balcony and he was also watching his father.

Her breath caught as she realised that Eli's son was close to the age their own baby would have been if things had been very different. It was also a reminder that Eli had a whole new life that not only didn't include her, it was on the other side of the world.

They had a past that had destroyed the trust they had once had with each other. Could an apology and amazing sex be all it took to wipe the slate clean?

How unlikely was that?

The medically fragile children at Camp Reki might be better equipped than most to handle this kind of shock because, sadly, most of them had dealt with the tragic loss of friends made during hospital admissions or members of the support groups they belonged to, but this was camp. Their happy place. The hardships and pain of real life were not supposed to intrude on their time here any more than was absolutely necessary to keep them safe and not disrupt their long-term treatments.

Maya didn't eat any breakfast herself. She moved from table to table, offering both children and their caregivers the opportunity to talk about how they were feeling and to have any questions answered. She was also offering hugs and encouragement to go to all the activities that they wanted to do today—both as distraction and to make the most of the fine weather. While the cyclone was still on course to bypass Reki Island, there was rain and some stronger winds forecast for the next few days.

Hazel was Maya's small shadow as she moved through the dining area and, while her trademark smile was as bright as ever, it was obvious that she was struggling. The blunt end of her arm, where a hand should have been, was constantly seeking the comforting touch of Maya's hand.

'Have you had any breakfast, sweetheart?' Maya asked.

'I'm not hungry.'

'Is that because you're feeling sad about Alice?'

Hazel's eyes filled with tears that overflowed as she nodded. Maya scooped her up into her arms and cuddled her.

'Why couldn't you make her better?' Hazel's voice was muffled against her shoulder.

'We tried,' Maya told her. 'We tried so hard. But Alice has been sick for a very long time and her poor, tired lungs had been having a hard enough time with just ordinary breathing. Having an asthma attack as well was too much for them.'

'Did it hurt?'

'No. She was asleep. I think she might have been dreaming about the pony ride she'd had because it made her so happy. She told us that it had been her best day ever.' Maya could feel tears gathering in her own eyes. 'And you know something?'

Hazel rubbed her nose on Maya's as she shook her head.

'Alice would want you to have the best day ever. Every day while you're at camp. What were you planning to do first this morning?'

'I'm supposed to be doing baking this morning. And dancing. And this afternoon is the scavenger hunt.'

'Ooh, I love scavenger hunts. Do you have any ideas about what you might have to find?'

'No.' But Hazel sounded more interested. 'Maybe a special sort of shell? Or flower?'

'Shall we go and see if we can find out any clues?'

Maya turned to walk towards the table near the door that was being set up to provide details for all the activities being offered for Day Six of this season's camp but she didn't move any further.

Because Eli, and Simon, were standing right in front of her.

Eli's glance told her that he was over any need for space. It was almost as if he was thanking her for having found a way to mention the elephant that had been in the room and, as he held her gaze, Maya felt her whole body start to tingle. It felt as though she was being held in his arms, not standing in front of him. As though he had the power, just by looking at her, to hold her upright. To give her strength?

This was not the time to think about the significance of what had happened between them last night or this morning. Or to try and see into the future. This was about taking everything, including what was likely to be a difficult day, one step at a time and, right now, Maya could be very grateful for this feeling of having someone by her side. Someone who cared enough to want her to be okay.

'Simon's planning to do the scavenger hunt, too,' he said. 'Can we come with you?'

Hazel wriggled out of Maya's arms. 'Yes,'

she said. 'We can do it together.' She smiled at Simon but he was staring up at his father.

Frowning.

Oh, help…

Had Simon sensed something in the way Eli and Maya had been looking at each other so intensely? Was it possible, when he'd been out on the balcony of the *bure*, that he had seen them kissing on the beach? She knew how protective Eli could be. If there was any chance of Simon being upset by Maya getting too close to his father, that would be the end of whatever seeds that might have been sown last night.

She tried to sound as if she was imparting a secret. 'I think Ana and Tevita will know all about what you're going to have to look for in the scavenger hunt. He might give you some clues and you can keep an eye out for things this morning.'

Hazel and Simon took off to the other side of the room to where Ana and her brother were unpacking boxes of small baskets that had cards attached to their handles.

'I heard some of what you said to Hazel about Alice,' Eli said quietly, as they followed the two excited children. 'Is she okay?'

'I think so. We need to support them and let them process things in their own way. How's Simon taking the news?'

'He didn't say much. Mike was in the clinic when we went in to do his factor infusion and they had a bit of a chat.' Eli shook his head. 'I think Si might have taken advantage of me wanting to make sure he was okay, though.'

Maya's steps slowed. 'What do you mean?'

'He said that he was feeling really sad about Alice but there was something that might make him feel better.'

'Which was?' They had both stopped walking, creating a human island in a room that was getting steadily busier.

'Being in the group that you're taking abseiling on the cliff this morning.'

Maya let out a huff of laughter. 'You didn't fall for that, did you?'

Eli grimaced. 'I kind of did.' His face softened as he caught her gaze again. 'Keep him safe for me? I've got a clinic this morning so I can't come and watch.'

He was asking *her* to keep Simon safe for him?

Wow...

It was almost like telling her that he could trust her again.

And that felt even bigger than being able to talk about the shared loss of their baby.

'I promise,' Maya said quietly. She couldn't

look away. 'And you know you can trust me. I never break a promise.'

The longing to be in his arms was so powerful it almost brought tears to her eyes. It was just as well they were in a crowded space and it would have been totally inappropriate to even think about touching each other.

The brush of skin on her hand didn't come from Eli, of course. And it was familiar enough to recognise without looking down—a gentle reminder that she was needed elsewhere.

'Okay, Hazel… I'm coming…'

Carlos was waiting outside the medical centre when Eli arrived.

'Are you not feeling well, Carlos?' Eli asked.

'I'm fine. But I'm going abseiling this morning and Maya said she wanted me to get a checkup.' Carlos shrugged. 'I guess she doesn't want me getting dizzy when I'm halfway down a cliff, which is fair enough.'

'No worries,' Eli said to Carlos. He was impressed with Maya's diligence in following up the dizzy spell Carlos had experienced at the airport when he'd first arrived. 'We'll do a quick check of your blood pressure and heart rate and rhythm and if they're okay you'll be good to go. Come on in—you'll be back with the group before you know it.'

A glance over his shoulder showed him the group, including Simon, gathering around Maya to put on their harnesses and other safety gear. He raised a hand and Simon waved back. They exchanged 'thumbs-up' signals.

Maya waved, too, and smiled. Eli went through the doors of the medical centre wrapped in the warmth of that smile. He could still see the look in her eyes when she'd promised to keep Simon safe. When she'd reminded him that he could trust her to never break a promise.

He knew he could trust Maya.

As much as he could trust himself.

He might have believed that trust had been broken but he'd been wrong, hadn't he?

Last night had proved that.

They had both been exhausted, physically and emotionally, having finally returned from such a heartbreaking day. They'd been deeply affected. Fragile enough to be utterly vulnerable. But when they were alone in Maya's *bure* there were no barriers to the comfort they could both give and receive because the solid foundation of that absolute trust was still there.

It hadn't changed.

It was also instantly recognisable. Eli had never found anything close to it with anyone else and he knew instinctively that it was a connection so rare he never would.

He would also never forget last night.

What was the dividing line, he wondered, between trust and love?

Was that what turned sex into making love?

Neither of them had said anything out loud last night but that was what they'd been doing, that was for sure.

Making love…

Oh, no… He couldn't let himself go any further down a mental track that had kept him awake for far too long after he'd finally gone back to his own *bure* in the early hours of this morning. He wasn't going to step back into a space that held the risk of heartbreak.

Because it wouldn't just be a risk for himself, would it?

Simon already thought Maya was amazing. Imagine if he and Maya did get back together. Simon would adore her. She'd be a mother to him and he'd have to worry that, one day, she might not come home from her work or a hobby like abseiling down cliffs and then he'd lose his mother all over again. It would be devastating for him.

Even if he didn't have Simon to put first in his life, Eli wasn't at all sure he could take that risk for himself. He certainly didn't have enough evidence that, despite giving in to the pull towards Maya, anything fundamental had really

changed to stop history ending up repeating itself. Last night was simply a product of having
gone through a traumatic and very emotional
experience together, combined with a past relationship that had made it too easy to get too
close, too quickly.

'Okay, Carlos. Sit on the side of the bed for
me and I'll take your blood pressure.'

Eli wrapped the cuff around the teenager's
arm and put the disc of his stethoscope on the
inside of his elbow, waiting to hear the sound
of the pulse starting and then finally fading as
he let the pressure out of the cuff. It was during those moments of silence that he could feel
that something was different about Carlos today.

'You okay, mate?' he asked quietly as he un-
wrapped the cuff. 'I know it's a bit of a tough
day for everyone.'

Carlos didn't respond, other than giving a
shrug. He lay quietly back on the bed when Eli
stuck on the sticky electrode patches needed to
monitor heart rate and rhythm for a few minutes
and then he suddenly spoke.

'She didn't want it.'

Eli raised his eyebrows.

'The lung transplant. We talked about it and
Alice told me she really didn't want it.' The
words were tumbling out now. 'She was so
scared of the pain and all the complications and

she said she didn't want to live longer if it might be even worse than it was now. She said she was sick of being sick. I'm glad she doesn't have to do it...that she's not scared any more.'

His voice broke and then he cleared his throat.

'There's nothing to stop me going to college, is there, Dr Peters?'

'No, not at all. There are lots of people out there who had heart transplants more than thirty years ago and the medicine to help, like new anti-rejection drugs and monitoring, is getting better all the time. There's nothing to stop you doing whatever you want to do with your life, Carlos, and every reason to go for it.'

'Do you think I could become a doctor? And help kids like Alice?'

Eli took a deep breath as he printed out a rhythm strip to go in Carlos's notes. It wasn't the first time a patient had given him pause for thought. When he looked up, he smiled at the courageous young man in front of him. It was his turn to clear his throat so that he could say something.

'I think you'll make a great doctor, Carlos. Now...your heart is behaving itself perfectly so how 'bout you get out there and do whatever it is that will make you feel better today?'

Carlos nodded. 'Thanks, Doc.'

'Any time.' Eli took the strip of graph paper

from the ECG monitor to attach to the patient notes as Carlos left the room, but for a long minute he found himself deep in thought.

Thinking about Carlos. And Alice.

About Simon and Sarah.

And Maya.

Life was precious. Too often, it was too short but the people who made the most of it and wanted to help others more than simply looking after themselves were the ones who made their time infinitely valuable.

People like Carlos.

And Maya.

Eli was aware of something else, too. He needed to be inspired by Carlos's attitude and let Simon follow whatever dreams he might have for his future.

Maybe he needed to think about his own future as well. He'd been so focused on his life with Simon that he hadn't realised what was missing. How lonely he was sometimes.

Until last night.

When he'd held Maya in his arms and realised just how much he had missed her. How much he still cared about her.

The weather began to change late that afternoon, with ominous-looking black clouds crowding the skies and the gusts of wind were strong enough for a warning to be issued not to go near the palm trees on the beach in case coconuts were falling. Not that anyone wanted to spend any more time on the beach today.

Tired children gathered in the main room before dinner to compare the contents of their scavenger hunt baskets. There were shells and pieces of coral, flowers and sticks and feathers amongst the natural objects and small plastic toys and wrapped candy treats that had been scattered around designated search areas by staff members. There was rather a lot of sand on the floor as well.

There had been a list of about twenty items printed on the laminated cards attached to the baskets but Hazel and Simon hadn't been able to get a heads-up on any of the items they might be searching for from either Ana or Tevita that morning.

'They could have told us *something*,' Simon complained as he spread the contents of his basket onto the floor in front of him. 'If I'd known we had to find a ginger flower I could have picked one this morning. There was a bush right beside the bottom of the cliff where we went abseiling, wasn't there, Maya?'

Maya and Hazel were sitting on the floor beside them.

'I should remember,' she said. 'Because they're

one of my favourite flowers, but I must have been too busy going up and down the cliff all morning to notice. There are ginger plants growing all over the island, though. Did it have long, spiky red flowers?'

'Yes. Just like the picture on the card of things we had to hunt for. I saw it when I was going up to the top of the cliff for my turn to come down with you. But I wasn't allowed to go back to the cliff by myself this afternoon and you weren't there to help, Dad.'

'No, I'm sorry, Si. Somebody cut their foot on a broken shell on the beach and we had to put some stitches in it. And someone else wasn't feeling very well so I wanted to keep an eye on them this afternoon. But you had lots of helpers, didn't you?'

'I guess…'

'I wish I could have come to watch you abseiling this morning, too. I've seen some of the photos.' They had been a bit hair-raising, to be honest. Simon had been halfway down a craggy cliff with his feet against lumps of sharp-looking volcanic rock, Maya hovering right behind him in her own harness. Maybe it was just as well he hadn't been there watching it. 'Was it scary?' he asked.

'Not really.' Simon shook his head. 'It was

just like the climbing wall, but Maya made me go really slowly.'

'We were just being careful,' Maya put in. 'It wasn't that slow.'

'It's always a good idea to be super-careful the first time,' Eli said. 'Sometimes you need to think twice about everything you do to make sure it's safe.'

Maya noticed the shell Simon was taking from his basket.

'That's a fabulous cowrie shell,' she said, touching its smooth, speckled brown surface. 'One of the biggest I've seen.'

'We had to find a big shell. And a curly one. And a piece of coral.'

'I got a big one with spikes,' Hazel said. 'See? I'm going to take it home and put it on my windowsill.'

'That's called a conch shell,' Maya told her. 'It's beautiful. And did you both find the secret I told you about—when I joked that you might really be going on a bear hunt?'

Simon laughed. 'You didn't say it was a *chocolate* bear.'

'I've eaten mine already,' Hazel said sadly.

'You can have mine.' Simon was tipping out the rest of his basket to find the small, foil-wrapped candy.

Eli leaned over to pick it up and pass it to

Hazel. He grinned at Maya. 'Did this come over from Australia with you, by any chance?'

'Yeah...so did the chocolate fish. They were my contributions to this year's scavenger hunt. We like to put different things in every year. The plastic geckos were Mike's choice this time.'

'How did you know the bear came from Australia?' Simon asked. 'And that it came with Maya?'

'It's a koala bear. They only come from Australia and that's where Maya lives now.'

Simon was staring at him. 'Where did she live before?'

'In New Zealand. Same as me. I told you about how I lived there for a while.'

The look Maya flashed at Eli felt like a question. Did Simon have any idea that they'd been more than friends?

Hazel broke a silence that had suddenly become a little awkward.

'Can I eat the bear now?' she asked.

'It's almost dinnertime, sweetheart,' Maya said. 'How 'bout you wait and have it for dessert?'

It was Simon who unknowingly answered that silent query that still seemed to be hanging in the air.

'Was Maya your girlfriend?' he asked.

'Um...' Eli caught Maya's gaze again. He was

trying to send a silent apology for opening what might be a can of worms but he was also searching for an indication of how private she wanted their past history to remain. If she wanted it to remain a secret, it would be a problem because he'd always been as honest with Simon as he was old enough to understand. About everything.

He'd never told him about having left a relationship when he'd come to look after Simon as a baby because it had never been relevant to their lives. It felt relevant now, however.

And...dangerous?

Was Maya deliberately not looking in his direction now? She was helping Hazel put her treasures back into her basket.

'We *were* friends,' Eli said uncomfortably, knowing that Simon was waiting for a response. 'It's a long time ago, Si.'

'Yes...' Maya got to her feet, still avoiding his gaze, picking up the basket as Hazel also got up a little awkwardly onto her prosthetic lower legs. 'You were a tiny baby, Simon—that's how long ago it was.' She handed the basket to Hazel, who hooked it over her elbow. 'We need to give your basket to Ana so she can count up how many things on the list you found. You might get a prize.'

Hazel bounced happily. 'I only had three things I couldn't find.'

'I only had one,' Simon muttered as he watched them walk away. 'That ginger flower.'

'You did well,' Eli said. 'I hope it was fun.'

Simon didn't say anything. He was giving Eli an odd look.

'What's up?' Eli asked. 'Are you feeling sad about Alice again?'

Simon started to nod but then shook his head.

'What is it, then?'

Simon ignored the question. He was silent as he piled his items back into the scavenger hunt basket but then his words came out in a rush. 'If you went to live in Australia, would you take me with you?'

Eli's jaw dropped. 'Why would I go and live in Australia?'

Simon's voice was no more than a mutter. 'Because that's where Maya lives.'

Oh, help… Was the electricity between himself and Maya, in the wake of their lovemaking last night, obvious enough that even an almost ten-year-old child could feel it? And feel threatened by it?

As if he would ever let anything come between him and this beloved child that had become the centre of his world.

Eli pulled in a breath. 'I'm not going to live in Australia,' he said firmly. 'But even if I went to live on the moon, Si, I wouldn't be leaving you behind. I would never leave someone I love so much behind. Why would you even think that?'

'Because…' Simon was brushing spilt sand together into a small pile on the floor. 'Because you're not really my dad, are you? You're only my uncle.'

'I adopted you, Si. You *are* absolutely my son.'

'It still doesn't mean that I'm your *real* son.'

Eli felt a shiver run down his spine. How—and when—had Simon even come up with such a notion? What had changed?

Nothing. Except they'd come here to this island.

And he'd, very unexpectedly, reconnected with Maya.

As if to underline Eli's sense of foreboding, there was a sudden flash of lightning from the dark clouds outside, a crack of thunder only seconds later and then the sound of torrential rain began to hammer on the roof.

Maybe that cyclone wasn't as far away as everybody had thought…

CHAPTER EIGHT

MAYA COULD SEE the slump of Simon's shoulders from the far side of the room and the way Eli was bent towards him as if they were having a very serious conversation.

She really hoped they weren't talking about her. Because neither of them looked happy and that was creating a cloud over any embryonic thoughts of this reconnection with Eli going any further. A stormy kind of cloud, even, like the ones that had gathered outside in the last couple of hours. The flash of lightning, followed too closely by a clap of thunder she could feel vibrating in her bones, made it seem as if the universe was issuing a warning not to pin any hopes on Eli wanting—or being available for—anything more than a short excursion down memory lane.

What was it he'd just said to Simon?

Oh, yeah…that it was always a good idea to be super-careful the first time and that you might need to think twice about everything you did to make sure it was safe.

Had he been thinking twice about the wisdom of getting too close to her when she'd seen him talking to Simon so seriously?

Maya didn't have the time to think about anything twice right now because she could see Mike near the doorway. It was the first time she'd seen him since this morning when he'd been flying out to be with Alice's family. Hazel was lining up with all the other children to get her dinner so Maya went out of the room to speak to Mike.

'How did it go?' she asked. 'I can imagine how rough the day's been.'

'Alice's parents are devastated,' Mike said. 'But I was very relieved that they're fully supporting Jake and the decision to let Alice come to camp. They're all on their way home now. I was glad I was there to make all the bureaucracy a bit easier for them.'

'You must be exhausted.'

'Can't afford to be,' Mike said. 'The weather was closing in as we flew back and I was fielding calls from the Fiji Meteorological Service. Cyclone Lily has started changing direction in the last sixty minutes. If it keeps going on its current trajectory, we might end up being a lot closer than we'd want to be. It could potentially make landfall on Reki Island.'

Maya's eyes widened. 'How severe is it now?

I heard that it got downgraded from a category four to a three earlier today.'

'It did. And they're hoping it might weaken further in the next few hours.'

'When's that expected to be?'

'Depends on how often the direction changes but we can expect heavy rain nine to twelve hours ahead of it making landfall and it looks like that's started already.'

'Did they give any idea of how long it will take to get past us?'

'Maybe twelve hours.'

'And it could get a lot worse out there than it is now.' Maya was frowning. A category five was the highest level for a tropical cyclone, but even at a three it could cause structural damage to buildings, ruin crops and damage trees.

'We need to be prepared for that,' Mike agreed. 'It's likely to blow through fast if it does reach us but I don't want to take any chances. Can you come with me to tick off the checklist and make sure that all our emergency kits are fully stocked at the medical centre?'

'Of course.'

'I've got ground staff out now, making sure that any outdoor equipment and furniture is secured or put away. Danny and James are getting the helicopter safely into the hangar. I'd better find Ana, too, before I do anything else. I'll call a meeting of all senior staff when everyone's had some dinner and Eli will need someone to stay with Simon.'

An hour later, however, it transpired that a babysitter would not be needed.

Mike and Maya had checked that all the medical kit backpacks in the medical centre were fully stocked and that drugs and IV fluids were still within their expiry dates when another call came in from the Meteorological Service. Cyclone Lily had changed direction again and they were now officially on standby for it making landfall on the island later in the evening. Mike had some big decisions to make.

'I want everybody to stay in the main complex overnight. These buildings were made to withstand a cyclone and we're on higher ground. It's not just the wind damage or flooding we have to anticipate, it's the storm surge. There are a lot of *bures* that are too close to the beach.'

Maya nodded. 'We don't want to be having to worry about getting medical care to the far corners of the resort either. We've got internal access to the medical centre from here and we don't have to worry about power failure, do we? We've got the solar power batteries and the generators.'

Mike nodded but let out a growling sound. 'I should have been more onto this. I was so focused on Alice's family today. We could have arranged ferries and evacuated people to the main island. We're going to have some scared kids on our hands and that's not going to help anyone who's physically fragile.'

'You didn't know,' Maya reminded him. 'As far as we knew, this cyclone wasn't going to come close enough to do more than give us a bit of stormy weather. By the time things changed it was already too late to evacuate anyone. You only just made it back here yourself.'

But Mike didn't look reassured. 'We've never had anything like this to deal with at camp. It's nowhere near cyclone season.'

'So let's try and make it exciting rather than scary for everyone,' Maya suggested. 'This can be the first ever camp sleepover. We'll move all the tables and chairs from the dining room and bring in their mattresses and bedding and any medical equipment they need. We can keep them entertained and keep everybody accounted for until the worst blows over.'

'Can I leave you to inform caregivers and start getting set up? Get Eli to help you? I need to get down to the village and let them know they can all come up here for shelter.'

'They may not want to leave their houses. Or their animals.'

'They could use the church as an evacuation

centre if they prefer. But they need warning about what's on the way—including the risk of a storm surge. I'll get a trailer loaded with supplies like bottled water and torches and take that down with a golf cart.'

Simon looked happier than he had all day.

'We're having a sleepover? All of us? In here?'

'Apparently so,' Eli said. 'It looks like this storm is going to get a bit worse before it gets better and this is the best building for us to be in.'

Several staff members were already clearing tables away to stack in another room and others could be seen outside, putting sandbags along the outside walls as extra protection. The heavy rain had stopped for the moment but, by the look of the clouds, another squall could come through at any minute.

'Stay here,' Eli instructed Simon. 'Ana and the others will be looking after you while we get set up. I think they're going to teach you some new songs, ready for our last night concert. I'm going to go back to our *bure* and get your pyjamas and toothbrush and stuff.'

'Are you coming to the sleepover, too?'

'Sure am.' Eli could see Maya opening one of the outside doors to this area. She had a raincoat on over her uniform but hadn't fastened it and a gust of wind nearly pulled it from her body as she stepped outside. She was trying to hold her hair out of her face with both hands and...

And Eli needed to be out there too. To find out where she was going and to make sure she was going to be safe.

'I'll be back really soon,' he told Simon.

He caught up with Maya as she passed the external entrance to the medical centre.

'Hey...where are you going?'

'I need to get a change of clothes that I can wear under protective overalls.' Maya's hair was whipping around her head in the wind. 'My steel-capped boots are under my bed, I think. And I need to find a hair tie and enough clips to stop my hair blinding me when I'm outside.'

A small frond from a palm tree hit Eli's shoulder and he heard the sound of something crashing onto the path ahead of them.

'What was that?'

'Probably a coconut. They're lethal in this kind of wind. I should have grabbed a hard hat before I came out. I'd better hurry.'

'I'm coming with you.' Eli put his arm around her shoulders, as if that was enough to protect her from whatever the rising wind could throw at them.

Maya grabbed what she wanted from her room and then they both ran back towards the main complex, but Maya slowed as they got closer. 'I need to get into our storage shed,' she told Eli.

He followed her in there and the roller door went up. The shed was lined with deep shelves and large enough to have a four-wheel all-terrain vehicle with a trailer attached parked in the centre of the space. He could see large items in the trailer, like a hard-shell basket rescue stretcher, coils of rope, blankets, tools like a chainsaw and shovel and…

'What are those metal things?' he asked.

'Struts,' Maya said. 'They're a fairly vital part of technical rescue equipment. For stabilising and lifting in case of someone being trapped under a collapsed building or a vehicle or something.'

She climbed onto the two-person seat of the ATV. 'I need to check that this is ready to go. Just in case.' She turned the engine on and revved it. 'Sounds good to go. Fuel tank's full. I'll leave the shed doors open.' Maya got off the bike to head to a rack where overalls were hanging. A shelf above the rack housed bright yellow hard hats with torches attached and a board to one side had portable radio transmitters hanging on hooks.

'I can't believe how well set up you are here,' Eli said. 'It must have cost a small fortune.'

'We've got sponsors that are happy to help

keep the camp running. And Mike fills in any gaps. This is his passion.'

'Have you got a pair of those overalls that would fit me?'

Her head turned sharply. 'You don't want to be out in a cyclone, Eli. It's dangerous. We'll need you in the medical centre if we run into any trouble. And Simon needs you nearby. I...' Maya sounded hesitant. 'I saw you talking to him after he asked you if I used to be your girlfriend. He... didn't look happy. Is everything okay?'

Maya wasn't looking happy either and Eli could feel a knot in his chest that was heavy enough to make it hard to take a breath. Without really thinking about what he was doing, he walked to Maya, took her in his arms and held her close.

He wasn't sure if this was intended to be an apology or he simply wanted her to know that, whatever happened next, he was never going to regret what had happened between them last night. When Maya lifted her chin to look up at him, he bent his head and kissed her softly. He lifted his head but then dipped it again to give her another kiss—he just couldn't help himself. Then he rested his chin against Maya's curls as he pulled her close again.

'I think Si might be feeling a bit confused,' he admitted. 'Threatened even, perhaps? He's never seen me in any kind of meaningful relationship so maybe he was a bit shocked by the idea I've had one in the past.'

'Oh, no…' Maya's eyes had widened.

'What?'

'I didn't think about it at the time but…it's just possible he might have seen us on the beach this morning. He might have heard the helicopter leaving and gone out to watch and then seen us talking and…'

'And kissing,' Eli finished for her. He let his breath out in a sigh. 'I'll have to explain that kissing someone doesn't automatically mean you're in a significant relationship.' He shook his head. 'I know he's old enough to realise how much things could change if there was someone else in our lives but…but he seems to have the crazy idea that I'd walk away from him if that *was* the case. He asked if I'd take him with me if I went somewhere else. Like Australia.'

'What?' Maya pulled back, looking shocked herself. 'Why on earth would he think you wouldn't?'

'I've always been honest with him. He knows he's adopted and that he's actually my nephew. I didn't think it mattered until he said something about not being my "real" son.'

He could read her thoughts in her eyes. She knew that Simon was the most important thing in his life and that he would never do anything to damage their relationship. He could see that she was dismissing the idea that she could ever be as important in his life as she had once been.

And he thought he could see—though it might be him projecting what felt almost like a fear of his own—that last night was already being parcelled away as a one-off. Something they probably shouldn't have done because it was a reminder of what they'd once had together but were never going to have again.

'It'll be okay,' Maya said quietly. 'He won't be upset if we're just friends. If we keep in touch after camp's over. Hey…maybe you could bring him out to Australia for a holiday some time. It's a brilliant country to visit.'

'And we'll be back for camp next year,' Eli added. 'If we get another invitation, that is.'

Maya smiled. 'I'll have a word with Mike. I don't think that'll be a problem.'

For a long moment, they held eye contact. As if they were letting go of what might have been, if things were different. As if Maya was trying to echo what he'd hoped he was silently communicating—that she had no regrets about last night.

It was Maya who broke the eye contact, turning away to pull down a pair of overalls. 'There's some bigger sizes on the other end of the rack,' she said. 'It's probably not a bad idea if you have some on hand. Just in case. You are the most highly qualified person here to deal with a trauma case if we get one.'

Above the noise of the wind outside, they could both hear something else. Someone calling.

'Help…we need help…'

Eli was right behind her as she ran outside. He recognised the big Fijian man as Sione—one of the gardeners at the resort. He had another man in his arms who was bleeding from a head wound and looked semi-conscious.

'Follow us.' Eli led the way to the medical centre. 'Can you tell us what happened?'

Maya flicked on the lights in the treatment room as Sione carried his friend Ma'afu to the bed.

'He was trying to get his boat out of the water,' he told them. 'I was running to help but a big wave caught it and he was underneath it when it came down on the beach.'

Eli was checking Ma'afu's airway and breathing, but when he put his stethoscope on his chest the injured man tried to push him away with a loud groan.

'Does that hurt?'

Ma'afu nodded.

'Does it hurt to breathe?'

He nodded again. Blood was running down

his face from the cut on his forehead and Maya grabbed a dressing and pressed it against the wound. 'Sione, could you hold this for me, please?' She took his hand and showed him how hard to press.

Eli was cutting Ma'afu's tee shirt to expose his chest and observe his breathing. If a lot of ribs were broken he might have a flail segment that would be visible and also a warning that his breathing could be significantly affected. The sharp ends of broken ribs could also cause bleeding that would accumulate in the chest cavity and affect the function of both the heart and lungs.

'Can we tilt the bed up to a forty-five-degree angle?' he asked Maya. 'And let's get some oxygen on. Ma'afu? If a really bad pain was a number ten and no pain at all was zero, what number would you give your pain at the moment?'

Sione had to shift his hand as he was translating the question, so that Maya could slip the elastic band of an oxygen mask over Ma'afu's head. With the bleeding now under control from the pressure, she could see the head wound was superficial. It would need stitches but that could wait.

'He says it's bad,' Sione reported. 'A number ten.'

Maya switched on the monitor beside the bed,

wrapped a blood pressure cuff around Ma'afu's arm and put a pulse oxygen clip onto a finger. Eli was gathering supplies to insert an IV line.

'I'm going to give you something for the pain,' he told their patient as he put a tourniquet around his arm. 'I know how painful it is for you to breathe at the moment. You'll feel better soon, I promise.'

They would also be able to do a secondary survey as soon as they had the pain at a more tolerable level. A thorough head-to-toe examination was a priority because there could well be other injuries to find.

'Are you allergic to any medications that you know of?' Eli asked.

Sione had to translate that question for Ma'afu and then he shook his head. 'He doesn't think so.'

As Maya stuck some electrodes onto his chest so they could watch his heart rate and rhythm, she watched Eli's swift, easy movements to insert the cannula, flush the line and then draw up and administer some morphine.

Sione reported that the medication had brought the pain level down to maybe a six and Eli topped the dose up a little.

'Do you want me to set up some fluids?' Maya asked him.

'Yes, please.'

An upward glance as Maya unravelled a giving set and pushed the spike into the port of a bag of saline revealed how focused Eli was on his task as he began the secondary survey, carefully examining Ma'afu's skull for any evidence of more damage than the laceration, like a skull fracture and potential brain injury. Then he shone a torch briefly into his eyes, checking for foreign objects like bits of shell or splinters and evidence of haemorrhage or an irregular iris shape, and swiftly moved to check their patient's ears for any sign of a CFS leak or blood. She knew he would be thinking ahead to any potential repercussions of the injuries that were already obvious and how they could handle them this far away from a fully equipped emergency department. They had no surgical facilities available and, for the moment, there was no backup of being able to evacuate a patient.

It was that familiar vertical line of utter focus between Eli's eyes that gave Maya a hard squeeze in her chest.

Or was it a tingle on her lips that clearly didn't want to let go of those kisses he'd given her so recently?

Whatever it was, it was enough to distract her from what she was doing for just a heartbeat as a wave of something that felt like sadness washed over her.

She still loved this man.

But it seemed as if their paths had crossed only to part again. Within a few days, they would be heading to opposite sides of the world.

That they could part as friends after so many years of unresolved pain they had caused each other should make it easier this time, shouldn't it? It was all Maya had been hoping for initially, after all. Was it only such a short time ago that the idea of anything more than friendship had been almost unthinkable? That taking the risk of being hurt again was too much to even consider?

Maya had the horrible feeling that walking away as friends might actually make it harder.

Not that this was the time to be thinking about it at all. Maya pushed it aside as she turned to check the current information they were receiving on the monitor screen.

'Sinus rhythm,' she said aloud. 'Tachycardia at one twenty.' The rate had increased. Was it because of a lack of oxygen? She pushed the button to inflate the automatic blood pressure cuff and as she waited for it to deflate again she couldn't help one more glance at Eli.

As if he felt the glance, he looked up to catch her gaze, unhooking his stethoscope earpieces. 'I'll top up the pain meds,' he said. 'And do an ultrasound.'

Had he heard diminished breath sounds? The

pounding of the rapid heart rate? He didn't need to tell Maya that he was concerned about internal bleeding that might be happening.

'What's the blood pressure?' Eli checked as he turned to set up the portable ultrasound machine. 'And oxygen saturation?'

The figures had just stopped changing on the screen.

'Blood pressure's dropped a bit. It's now one zero five over sixty. SpO2 is ninety-five.'

He caught her gaze again, just for a heartbeat, and she knew they were thinking the same thing—that it was now urgent for them to find out whether there was enough blood or air, or both, in the chest cavity to impede the function of the lungs or heart.

Them...

Part of that silent communication had made Maya feel that they were doing this together, as a team, and there was a poignancy there that reminded her too much of having been a team in their personal lives as well.

Was Eli feeling that, too? Was that why he sounded so professional as he put some gel on the side of Ma'afu's chest and got Sione to translate the reason he was doing this examination.

'It will let us see even a small amount of bleeding. An ultrasound can detect small amounts of bleeding far better than an X-ray. As little as ten mils—that's only two teaspoons. You'd need at least a hundred mils for it to show up on an X-ray.'

'What will you do if he is bleeding inside?' Sione asked.

'We'd put a tube in to take the blood away and make it easier for Ma'afu to breathe well. Can you ask whether this is hurting him?'

Thanks to the pain medication, it didn't seem to be too painful for the probe of the ultrasound to be positioned on the right side where the ribs were fractured, above the liver and just under the diaphragm. Maya watched as Eli angled it up to see into the thoracic cavity. He sensed that she was also watching the screen.

'That's the liver in the middle of the screen,' he said quietly. 'And that white line is the diaphragm. You can see it moving with each breath. And that dark patch there beside the liver? Can you see that?'

'Yes. Is that fluid?'

'Yes.' Eli moved the probe to examine the area more closely. 'Blood.'

'What's the odd-shaped bit that's waving?'

'Part of the lower lobe of the lung. It's compressed into that shape by the pressure of the amount of blood that's collecting.' Eli put his hand on Ma'afu's arm. 'We do need to put a tube into your chest,' he told him. 'I'm going to give you some local anaesthetic so it doesn't hurt, but you might feel some poking and pushing. Sione, can you help him stay as still as possible, please?'

'Yes, of course.'

'And, Maya? I'll need your assistance.'

'Of course.' Her words were an echo of Sione's agreement but they felt as if they were saying much more.

That Eli could ask her for anything and she would be there, by his side, without hesitation. Even if it had nothing to do with a professional situation like this. A tiny piece of her heart was breaking as she remembered how unlikely it was that he would ask.

She watched Eli's hands as he swiftly identified the landmarks he needed, like the tip of the scapula and the line of the twelfth rib to mark where the diaphragm was. Maya prepped and draped the skin and Eli worked fast, making a small incision and doing a blunt dissection and making a track for the tube that he inserted carefully, held in the teeth of a clamp.

Maya had the suture ready for Eli to secure the tube, with stitches in the skin and multiple knots, before winding the suture around the tube and making more knots. They covered the area with a gauze dressing, taped into place. Blood was already collecting in the drainage bottle hanging on the side of the bed.

'All done,' Eli told their patient. 'Well done for staying so still. We want you to rest now, okay?'

Ma'afu was drowsy. 'Thank you,' he mumbled beneath his mask.

Within a short time his vital signs were improving, with oxygen levels increasing and his heart rate slowing. By this time, other staff members were gathering in the medical centre and were ready to take over monitoring Ma'afu's condition.

When Maya left the treatment room to dispose of the soiled drapes, she found Mike had just returned from his visit to the village. He had a portable radio clipped to his belt.

'I've left a radio with Petero in the village,' he said. 'He'll call if there's any problems. We're on channel three.'

Maya nodded. Pete was another one of the groundsmen at the resort, a friend of Sione's and just as sensible and reliable. He was a good choice as the village contact.

'I'll go and get a radio for myself so I'm in the loop,' she said.

The rain had started again and the wind was getting strong enough to be howling across the roof. A gust was almost enough to knock Maya off her feet as she headed back to the storage shed and she felt an apprehensive shiver run down her spine. This storm was coming in harder and faster than they'd expected. She could only hope it would blow past and dissipate just as quickly.

Dressed in her overalls and boots, Maya had no sooner turned on another fully charged radio and set it to channel three when she heard a panicked voice.

'Mike… Mike… Can you hear me?'

'I'm here, Pete.' Mike's voice was calm. 'You're coming through loud and clear. What's happened?'

'It's a tree…' The radio crackled. It sounded as if there were people screaming in the background. 'It's come down on a house. We can't get in and…and I think there might be people inside.'

Maya pushed the button on her radio. 'I heard that, Mike. I'll head to the village straight away. Pete? Can you hear me? Pete…?'

There was a crackling sound loud enough to make any words incomprehensible. And then it stopped. Mike's voice came through to break the ominous radio silence.

'Go and see what we need to deal with, Maya. But be careful, okay? I'll get a team on standby for backup.'

Maya clipped the radio to her pocket and

reached for a hard hat. She started the ATV and was driving it out of the shed when she had to stop.

Eli was right in front of her.

'You're not going there alone,' he said. 'I'm coming too.'

CHAPTER NINE

IT WAS A NO-BRAINER.

Simon was safe. He was inside. Tucked up in a building designed to withstand the destructive force of a tropical cyclone, with a thick cushion of sandbags as extra protection against a possible storm surge. There were any number of people available to keep him safe.

Maya was about to head out into the storm and put herself in danger to help others.

Alone.

Eli couldn't have stayed in the safety of the resort, knowing that Maya was out there in danger. He had to go with her.

It would be too hard to stay in safety here and imagine what might be happening because that would tap into too many memories.

Of being at home and hearing the news that his parents had been killed in that avalanche.

Of being in New Zealand when Sarah had been so badly injured.

It was possibly a timely reminder that he didn't

want to go back to where he had to live with that kind of fear on a regular basis but he was here and this was a crisis and...

And it was almost as if he could try and make up for not being anywhere near the people he had loved, and lost, in the past.

He might not be able to prevent disaster but at least he wouldn't be able to beat himself up for not being there.

And having made sure the island villagers had shelter and supplies and a means of contact, Mike needed to stay in the medical centre and near all the children and their caregivers that he had taken responsibility for when he'd accepted them into this camp for children with complex medical needs. There were plenty of medical staff who could care for the only, now stable, casualty so far but there could well be others in the village and Eli was the most highly qualified medic on the island to deal with traumatic injuries. Another no-brainer.

He kept Maya waiting for less than a minute, grabbing a radio, dragging on a pair of overalls made of strong protective fabric to cover the clothes he was wearing and jamming a hard hat on his head after he climbed on board the ATV, fastening the strap as they took off down the track that led to the village. The sheets of water from the torrential rain were being driven off the visors of their helmets by the wind but the visibility was still only a few metres ahead at most and the further they went from the resort, the rougher the track became.

Eli had to hand it to Maya. She could handle this vehicle with apparent ease and she was taking them to where they were needed as fast as possible. There were safety belts but Eli still needed to hang onto the bar of the anti-roll protection frame to try and stop himself bouncing against Maya when they hit any bumps or potholes. This should have been terrifying but, strangely, it wasn't. Not only because he was so focused on what they were heading towards.

It was also because he had complete faith in Maya.

She'd been doing this kind of thing for years. She knew what she was doing, and she wasn't about to take any stupid risks. This had nothing to do with an adrenaline junkie who was looking for thrills. This was a courageous woman who was prepared to put her own safety at risk because others were in danger.

He was proud of her.

Okay…he hadn't coped that well with the background anxiety of her working in a profession that could put her in danger and, worse, having hobbies that were even riskier, but that was because it tapped into the tragic loss of his parents at a vulnerable time in his life and how protective he'd been of his sister afterwards and that mistrust of tempting fate had continued, thanks to being reinforced by the accident victims he treated in the emergency department who hadn't been careful enough.

But Maya had been right when she'd said simply that 'accidents happen'. That she hadn't been to blame for what had caused the tragic loss of their unborn baby.

Mike had said something similar in that introductory staff meeting.

'Accidents or unexpected medical events can happen any time or anywhere...'

He'd always known how much he could trust Maya—right from the first moment he'd met her.

But had he pushed that knowledge away so many years ago? Had it been buried by the fear that the worst was happening? Had allowing himself to ignore that faith in Maya contributed to the way they'd been pushed apart by events and emotions spiralling out of control? And was it why, despite finding each other again, it felt as if it could be too late to undo enough of the damage that had been done ten years ago? Or was the real problem that there were new barriers to them being together?

Like a boy on the cusp of adolescence who didn't feel secure enough?

It was just as well that Maya had instantly understood the implications of Simon asking if Eli would go to Australia without him. That she had made it clear that she believed their night together had been no more than a one-off. For old times' sake.

He'd always loved the way they could communicate silently like that.

And that she'd always had his back.

A snapped branch bouncing off the roll bars of the quadbike, catching his helmet as it dropped, was enough to jolt Eli's thoughts back to the present.

'You okay?' Maya had to shout to be heard over the shriek of the wind.

'Glad I'm wearing a helmet.'

'We're almost there.'

The small church was the first building they got to. Sturdily built, it was where the villagers were gathering for shelter and there were people holding torches and carrying armloads of supplies heading inside. Others were waiting for this help to arrive and they ran beside the vehicle as Maya kept going.

'This way…this way…!' they yelled.

There were *bures* still standing but on the edge of the village an enormous tree had come down, crushing a house beneath it.

'Whose house is it?' Maya asked. 'Is anyone missing?'

'We can't find Tevita.' Pete, the groundsman who'd made the call for help, was here. He'd managed to push into a section of the foliage but there were thick branches blocking him from getting any further. 'I've called someone at the resort to see if he went to find Ana, but someone else thought he was with his grandparents, Lani and Josefa, helping them pack what they needed to go to the church. We can't find them either. They never made it to the church. And… this is their house.'

The tree was massive, a Pacific kauri that was probably over a hundred years old. It had been growing on the outskirts of the village but it was tall enough for the mass of foliage and branches on the top of a clean trunk to totally engulf the house.

The headlights of the quadbike were shining on broken branches creating sharp barriers within a mass of the leathery, dark foliage. Or were they the beams that might have been holding up the roof of the *bure*?

'I've got a chainsaw in the trailer,' Maya told him.

Pete had it going only minutes later. He started cutting sections of branches and there were willing hands to carry the logs away. These were people without any protective clothing or hard hats on and they should be seeking shelter in the church with the other villagers, but how could Eli order them away?

There were people they loved somewhere under that tree, potentially injured amongst the wreckage of their home.

And one of them was a boy who wasn't much older than Simon.

'What can I do?' Eli asked Maya. 'How can I help?'

More people had gathered, including Jackie, one of the nurses from the medical centre, who held a raincoat around herself as she braced against the relentless wind and rain.

'Mike said to tell you that Ma'afu's doing well.' She had to raise her voice above the noise of the extreme weather and the chainsaw being used. 'The bleeding has slowed down and his breathing is better. The oxygen levels are almost normal.' She watched Maya fastening the knee pads around her legs. 'Do I need some of those?'

Maya shook her head. 'It's not safe out here,' she told her. 'You can be more help by going into the church and looking after anyone in there who's injured. I imagine there's quite a few people with cuts and bruises by now. We're trying to carve a passage through the tree branches to get to this house and I'll probably need to crawl so that's why I need the pads. I've got Eli here if we need to treat anybody, but if you find anything you're not comfortable to deal with yourself, send someone to let us know and he can come and help.'

'Take one of the first aid kits for now,' Eli added, handing her a small backpack. 'There are plenty of bandages and dressings in here.'

'Where's the church?'

Maya could see someone she recognised coming towards them, leaning into the gusts of wind.

'Timi can show you.'

But Timi had something to say first. 'They're in the church,' he said. 'Lani and Josefa.'

'Oh, thank goodness for that. Are they okay?'

'Josefa has cut his hand, that's all.'

'Take Jackie back to the church with you. She can look after him. What about Tevita?'

Timi shook his head. 'They don't know where he is. Lani thinks he might have gone to try and find Ana at the resort.'

The sound of the chainsaw stopped as Timi and Jackie turned to run back down the track. Pete emerged from the remaining foliage a few seconds later.

'I can see into part of the house,' he told them. 'But I can't get closer. There are big branches that come straight from the trunk and if I cut there might not be enough to stop it all coming further down onto the house.'

'It's good that you stopped,' Maya said. 'We may not need to do any more here. Josefa and Lani are safe at the church.'

'Are they?' Pete looked surprised. 'When I stopped the chainsaw, I thought I could hear someone calling. Maybe it was the wind?'

Or maybe it was Tevita.

Maya radioed Mike to update him on the situation and to ask if there'd been any sign of Tevita at the resort.

'No,' he said grimly. 'Ana thinks he would have stayed with his grandparents.'

'He might be trapped in the house, then,' Maya said. 'I'll have to go and have a look. We can't give up until we know where he is.'

'Be careful…' Mike sounded worried.

'Roger that.'

Maya tightened the strap on her hard hat and clipped her radio back to her belt.

Looking up to make sure Eli also had his radio, she caught the look on his face.

The fear…

For her?

It gave her heart a squeeze that hurt. But it also gave her a strength that was more than she could ever have found on her own.

'I know what I'm doing,' she reassured him. 'I've done a lot of search and rescue training.'

Not that it had covered an event precisely like this, but she had learned about how to approach a building collapse or other situations where the safety of rescuers depended on the stability of structures or vehicles. Maybe the branches of this enormous tree were working like the struts that protocols might have called for and they would keep her safe.

Oddly, it did feel safer as she went into the tunnel Pete had created. It was suddenly a little quieter in here. More sheltered. But it was still frightening. She could hear the creaking of the branches high above her and feel the snap of something breaking under her boots. At any moment she knew she might hear the cracking sound of a huge branch unable to take the weight of what it was supporting and it was highly unlikely she would have enough time to avoid being crushed. She glanced behind her, to reassure herself that she had an escape available, but what she saw was anything but reassuring.

'Eli…what are you *doing*?'

She didn't want Eli to be involved in what could be an unpredictably dangerous action. It was unthinkable to imagine him being seriously injured. Killed, even?

'Go back,' she ordered sharply. 'I have no idea how safe this is.'

'Keep going,' was all he said. 'There's no time to waste.'

But she hesitated for just another heartbeat. Because she remembered the fear she'd seen in his eyes only moments ago. The fear for her safety. The fear she was feeling for him because...because she loved him *this* much.

Did this mean that Eli loved her that much, too?

The thought barely formed before it was gone. They both heard the faint cry of someone calling for help.

'Tevita?' Maya pushed forward. She got to the big branch that Pete had told her about, but she could see that there was enough of a gap to squeeze underneath it. Just. Then there were smaller branches to push past and she felt one of them flick back against her cheek hard enough to make it sting. There was something different underfoot now, however, and the torch on her helmet showed her that it was the thick, thatched plant material used for the walls and roofs of the local *bures*. Ahead of her, amongst more broken pieces of thatched panels, she could see the colours of a flower-patterned fabric and it looked like a sarong being used as a bedcover. Beside the mattress, hunched on the ground, she

could see the lanky limbs of a boy barely into his teens, his face tear-streaked and completely terrified, but at least he was conscious and alert.

'Tevita…' She was beside him in moments. 'It's okay…we're going to get you out of here.'

She needed to check that he wasn't hurt, but she took a moment to put her arm around his shoulders to comfort him because she could see him shaking with fear. 'It's okay,' she said again. 'Eli's here too.'

He was. Right here beside them, and it almost felt as if he'd put his arm around her shoulders.

'Does anything hurt, Tevita?' Eli asked.

Tevita nodded. 'My leg,' he said. 'I can't move it. I fell over when…when the tree came down.'

He had his leg bent and his lower legs were bare beneath his shorts. Maya could see a large, distinct lump on one side of it.

'Looks like he's dislocated his patella,' she said. 'I don't think it's a knee dislocation, though. There's no gross deformity of the knee joint.'

Eli nodded. He was using his torch to scan the rest of Tevita's body as well, however. 'Did you hit your head?' he asked.

'No.'

'Can you take a deep breath? Does it hurt?'

'No.'

'What about your tummy?'

'It's just my leg. It really hurts…'

'Can you wriggle your foot?'

'No.'

'Can you feel me touching it?'

'Yes.'

Maya caught Eli's gaze. 'We can't move him with his leg bent and knee locked like this.'

'Let's give him some pain relief and see if we can reduce it.'

Maya opened the pack to find what she needed as Eli explained to Tevita what they were going to do.

'You've dislocated your kneecap,' he said, 'which means it's in a place that's stopping you from being able to move your leg. We're going to put it back by straightening your leg.'

'No...' The sound was almost a sob. 'That will hurt even more.'

'Maya's getting something ready for you that will stop it hurting too much. And it will feel a lot better afterwards. We have to be quick, though, Tevita. It's not safe for any of us in here. Can you be brave and help us?'

Maya glanced up to see that Eli had his hand on Tevita's shoulder and the boy's gaze was fixed on his. She could almost feel the bond of trust that had somehow been created between the two of them in the space of such a short time.

'Yes...' Tevita said.

Maya had poured methoxyflurane into the

base of an inhaler. 'We call this a green whistle,' she told Tevita. 'You breathe in and out with your mouth on the green bit and it won't hurt when we straighten your leg. Okay? It won't take long.'

Tevita nodded. He closed his lips around the mouthpiece of the inhaler and breathed in cautiously. The second time he took a deeper breath.

Maya looked at Eli. 'Ready?'

He nodded. He held Tevita's lower leg while she palpated the edge of the patella.

'On your count,' Eli told her.

'Suck hard on the whistle,' Maya advised Tevita. She waited until he was taking a really deep breath of the analgesic. 'On three,' she said to Eli. 'One…two…*three*…'

Eli lifted Tevita's foot to straighten his leg. As he did so, Maya pushed the side of the patella to shift it back to the front of the knee where it belonged.

'Take another big breath, Tevita. You're doing really, really well…'

She lifted it slightly to help it over the ridge on the end of the femur and she could feel the clunk as the dislocation was reduced.

'Ooh…' The sound Tevita made was one of relief. 'That feels better.'

'We're going to put a bandage on it,' Eli told him. 'And then we're going to get you out of here. You'll need an X-ray to make sure you haven't broken any of the bones in your knee.'

The sound of something cracking overhead reminded them that the sooner they were out of here, the better. There was no time to try and get better access and use a stretcher but, with his leg straightened and the knee well bandaged, Tevita was able to crawl and they got him out of the wreckage of the house and into the foliage of the tree. It was harder getting under the big branch but there were others in the tunnel now, wanting to help. Eli had radioed Pete to get the scoop stretcher from the trailer and once Tevita was inside it they could slide him out the rest of the way with ease.

They got out into clear space to find that the wind had dropped noticeably and the rain was much lighter.

'It could be the eye of the cyclone,' Eli said. 'Which might mean it'll pick up again soon, but this is good. We can get Tevita to the medical centre.'

Strong men were waiting to lift the stretcher and put it into the back of a four-wheel drive station wagon from the village. Tevita's grandfather was already in the vehicle, his bandaged hand in a sling.

'You go with them,' Maya suggested to Eli, when they'd loaded the stretcher. 'I'll drive the

ATV back when I've checked on how Jackie's going in the church. I need to find out whether anyone else is unaccounted for. This will be the best time to look for them if we need to.'

But Eli shook his head. 'I'll come with you. Mike's on standby to give Tevita an X-ray and check for any other injuries so I'm not needed there at the moment. I don't want you driving anywhere by yourself. We can't know if or when the wind's going to get worse again. Or how bad it's going to be.'

It was over an hour later that they left the church. Every one of the villagers had been checked. Some superficial wounds had been cleaned and dressed. They made sure that people who had conditions like diabetes, asthma or heart problems had any medication they might need on hand. Jackie would stay with the group until morning. Both she and Pete had radios to call for help if they ran into any trouble.

People were anxious but none of them wanted to leave their village and go to the resort for shelter. They were in a well-built, solid structure and they had mattresses and blankets and food and, most importantly, each other. There were animals being kept safe as well. Pet dogs and chickens in crates.

'Where are the ponies?' Eli asked. 'Are they safe?'

'They've been through storms before,' Pete told him. 'Their paddocks are tucked in behind the mountain and they know where to find the best shelter. We'll go and check on them as soon as it's safe. This might get worse before it gets better but I have a feeling it will have all blown over by morning.'

'Let's hope so,' Eli said.

'Call if you need us,' Maya said. 'I'll come back at first light tomorrow, but are you okay for us to go back to the resort now? I think that Simon will be wanting to see that his dad is safe and we both want to check on how Ma'afu's doing.'

'Go.' Pete nodded. 'We'll be fine. Go now, before it gets any worse out there.'

They climbed into the ATV and it was only then, as a fresh gust of wind swept Maya's hair away from her face, that Eli saw the streak of dried blood on her cheek, near her ear.

Oh, *man*...

That knot in his gut that formed faster than the speed of light at the thought of Maya being injured. It should have been a warning but it was too late, wasn't it? He'd known he still cared deeply about her—okay, *loved* her—but he'd shied away from the idea of being *in* love with her so successfully it hadn't occurred to him that it had happened all over again. In fact, he realised, it probably hadn't.

This felt too familiar.

It felt like coming home.

He'd never *stopped* being in love with her, had he?

Whatever had buried that intensity of how he felt about her had simply disappeared. Blown away by the same deadly winds that had blown the tree down onto the house they'd just crawled into together?

'You've hurt yourself,' he exclaimed, reaching up to touch Maya's face.

'It's nothing. Just a scratch.'

But he didn't take his hand away. He leaned closer.

'We should get going,' Maya said. 'Simon needs you.' But she didn't start up the quadbike. She was leaning into his hand, turning her face so that it was cupped in his fingers. She was looking up at him at the same time and it was a look that he could have fallen into if he let himself.

He wanted to tell her that he still loved her.

He wanted to tell her that everything was going to be okay and that they would find a way through this but, right now, it was more important that they got going. They needed to get back to the safety of the resort before the wind and rain picked up again. This was something he could actually do to keep Maya safe.

He took just a moment, however, to grab what could be the only time they might have alone together for a while.

To do this…

To kiss her with a fierceness that might let her know just how much he loved her.

She was kissing him back with a need that felt tinged with something poignant. Sadness, even?

He knew why. He'd felt the tacit agreement that this couldn't be allowed to mean too much when Simon was going to need his dad more than ever as he approached adolescence. When he was already feeling insecure.

No…he couldn't promise that everything was going to be okay, could he?

Not yet…

CHAPTER TEN

ELI SCRAMBLED OUT of the ATV as soon as Maya pulled it to a standstill outside the doors of the medical centre as they got back to the resort.

'I'll be back to join the medical team in a minute,' he said. 'I just need a moment to check on Simon first.'

Maya nodded. Of course he did. She saw him running to the main dining room and conference area that made the U shape around the swimming pool. It was late enough for all the children to be asleep by now but Simon might well still be awake, worried about his father being out in the storm.

While the strength of the wind and rain had increased since they'd left the village, it didn't feel quite as frightening as it had earlier this evening. Was it subsiding into a tropical storm rather than a cyclone? Was she simply getting used to it?

The way she was getting used to the idea that she and Eli could never be more than friends?

That kiss they'd just shared, though…

It hadn't felt like it was coming from nothing more than friendship.

But maybe that was just wishful thinking.

What was it that Eli had said when she'd told him that Simon might have seen them kissing on the beach?

Oh, yeah…

'Kissing someone doesn't automatically mean you're in a significant relationship…'

Seeing Mike through the window of the treatment room, Maya tapped on the door and went inside. Mike was working alone, stitching the cut on Josefa's hand. He glanced up briefly.

'All good?'

'Yes. We've left Jackie and Pete in charge at the village and they've both got radios so they can contact us. Everyone's accounted for, either in the church or here at the resort, and I said I'd go back at daybreak to check on them. I have a feeling that the worst will be over by then.'

Mike nodded. 'Yes…the latest report from the Meteorological Service has downgraded Cyclone Lily to a tropical storm. We're still waiting to see what the storm surge will be like at high tide and we don't want anyone outside sightseeing first thing tomorrow. Okay, Josefa…that local anaesthetic should be working by now. Can you feel me touching your hand?'

'No.'

Mike picked up a suture from the tray beside him, taking another glance at Maya at the same time.

'You okay? What's happened to your cheek?'

'It's nothing. Just a scratch. I'm good.'

'I heard about you rescuing Tevita from under the tree.' Mike was carefully inserting a stitch below skin level in the deep cut Josefa had at the base of his thumb. 'Well done, you. And Eli.'

The swift glance was a silent question. Had she been okay, working under such fraught conditions with someone that she might find it difficult to be that close to?

Maya's smile was intended to reassure him. She was strong. She could handle this.

'How's Ma'afu?' she asked.

'Sore, but breathing pretty well. We've done an X-ray to check that the chest drain is in the best place—and it is. Eli did a good job. He's got a few broken ribs, but the internal bleeding seems to have stopped. We'll need to keep a careful eye on him until we can transfer him to hospital. We've cleaned up his head wound but we're watching for any signs of concussion or TBI.'

'And Tevita?'

'He's also had an X-ray. He's lucky—he seems

to have escaped getting an osteochondral fracture. Ana's in with him now.'

'She's a good girl,' Josefa put in. 'She's been like a mother to him since they came to live with us here.'

'I remember when that happened. It was our first year of holding the camp.' Five years ago, when Josefa and Lani's only daughter, a single mother who'd been living in Suva, sadly died.

Five years but it felt like yesterday. It was ten years since she'd felt as if she had a future with Eli but that, too, suddenly felt as though she'd only just lost sight of it. She could feel that loss all over again.

Because of that kiss?

Mike was closing the wound at skin level now, with a few neat sutures. Maya picked up the package holding a sterile dressing and peeled it open so Mike could take it when the last suture had been placed and knotted.

Mike was doing exactly that when there was a tap on the door of the treatment room and it was opened enough for Eli to peer in. His hair was wet enough to be dripping water. Why had he been outside when he could get from the conference area to the medical centre through an internal corridor?

Something didn't feel right.

'Sorry to interrupt,' Eli said. 'But you haven't seen Simon around here, have you?'

Maya's heart skipped a beat at the note in Eli's voice. 'Wasn't he with all the other kids?'

'No.' Eli sounded like he was determined to stay calm. 'He wasn't on his mattress or in the bathroom. Carlos said he hadn't seen him since they all had a game of balloon football in the dining room, before the movie started, but he remembered that he asked one of the camp crew if he knew where I was. Carlos thought he might have come here to see if I'd got back from the village but he's not in the waiting room or the office.'

'Could he have gone to your *bure*?' Maya suggested.

'I'll go there next. I wouldn't have thought he'd want to go out into that weather, though.' He sucked in an audible breath. 'I'd better find Ana. She might know something.'

'She's with Tevita,' Mike told him. He smoothed the dressing on Josefa's hand and picked up a gauze bandage. 'Go with him,' he said quietly to Maya as Eli disappeared. 'He needs you.'

Ana was horrified to learn that Simon wasn't with the other children.

'He was there when I got the news that Tevita and Grandpapa were being brought here.

He promised he'd go straight to bed after they had the hot chocolate and marshmallows that the chefs were making for everyone.' Ana had tears gathering in her eyes. 'I shouldn't have left him. I'm so sorry…'

'You needed to be with your family,' Eli told her. 'This isn't your fault, Ana. Simon knew where he was supposed to be. I don't understand why he made a promise he didn't keep. What was he doing when you last saw him?'

'He'd just finished watching the movie they'd put on in the dining room and he'd been sorting through his scavenger hunt basket again. He was kind of disappointed that he hadn't found everything on the list, you know? He thought he might have won a prize if he had.' Ana bit her lip. 'I think he wanted something special to show you, Dr Peters. He always tries so hard at everything because he wants you to be proud of him.'

Eli felt a chill run down his spine.

The pieces were suddenly coming together.

The fragments of old fears had morphed into the birth of new ones. The need to protect the people he loved and the guilt of not having done it well enough.

And every piece had something to do with Maya, didn't it?

It had been Maya who had persuaded Eli to let Simon do the climbing activities he wanted to do. Not just on the relatively safe climbing wall but on a real cliff.

Simon might have seen him kissing Maya on the beach.

He'd definitely heard that panicked message come across the radio about the tree coming down on a house and he'd listened to his father telling him that he had to go with Maya because people might be hurt and she might need him to help her. He'd left without a backward glance, hadn't he? He'd gone to try and protect Maya when he should have stayed here and looked after Simon.

Had Simon been worried that he'd been left behind? Had he somehow convinced himself that an old girlfriend might be more important than a son who didn't feel 'real' and could therefore be left behind for ever? That if Eli could leave him behind at camp so easily, maybe he *could* leave him behind to go as far as Australia?

The prospect of being abandoned would have been even more frightening in the middle of a storm.

Eli turned to Maya. She was pale. Her eyes were reflecting his own fear that he was desperately trying to control.

His voice sounded hollow. 'He might have tried to follow us to the village. He knew that was where I was going with you.'

'I'll get Mike,' she said. 'We'll find him, Eli...'

He started to follow her but had to pause to take a ragged breath. The fear was getting harder to control.

Maybe Simon hadn't gone looking for him at all. Had he, in fact, run away in a different direction because he was convinced that Eli wanted to be in a relationship with Maya again? That he might be in the way?

Why hadn't he taken the time to reassure him properly?

Simon had been his priority since the moment he'd picked him up into his arms after he'd arrived back in London to be by Sarah's bedside. Since he'd promised his sister that he would always look after her precious baby.

Nothing could be allowed to come between himself and Simon.

Not even Maya.

And the only thing that mattered right now was to find Simon.

'I'll contact Pete,' was the first thing Mike said as came out of the treatment room. 'He can start looking around the village. I'll get people here to search the resort.' He held Eli's gaze. 'You need to check your *bure* and...' He was frowning now. 'If he's not there, check the beach. It's close to your *bure* and it's possible that Simon couldn't find his way in the dark. We need to make sure

202 PARAMEDIC'S REUNION IN PARADISE

he's nowhere near the waves that might come in at high tide.'

'I'll come with you,' Maya said.

But Eli was already turning away. This was his son. His responsibility. He couldn't let himself be distracted in any way. How could he try and protect Maya and Simon at the same time without being torn in two, knowing how he felt about Maya but knowing that he had to do what was best for Simon?

It was only the commanding tone in Mike's voice that made him turn back.

'Don't go alone,' he ordered. 'Take Maya with you.'

It felt like Eli didn't want her to be here with him.

If she let it, it might feel as if the last ten years had been peeled away to reveal that she was still in love with Eli but he didn't feel the same way, but the fear that she could be facing the same rejection that had nearly destroyed her all those years ago had to be pushed aside. This was about Simon. A gorgeous boy with an adventurous spirit and so much courage. A vulnerable child who might well be in danger.

They *had* to find him.

There was no sign that he had gone to the *bure* he'd been sharing with Eli.

'Nothing's been touched since we came in here to get the things he'd need for the sleepover,' Eli said. 'If he *was* looking for me, he would have come here or to the medical centre.'

'Or tried to get to the village,' Maya added. 'Except...'

'What?' The prompt to continue was sharp.

'It was what he was doing when Ana last saw him.'

'Looking through that basket? Being disappointed that he wasn't going to get a special prize for finding everything in the scavenger hunt?' Eli's voice was raw. 'So that I'd be proud of him and not leave him behind when I went off to Australia with you...'

'We'll find him,' Maya promised, even though she knew she had no right to be so sure. 'What if he's gone off to try and find that ginger flower? So he could get that recognition? The cliff's not that far away.'

'I don't even know where it is.' Eli sounded angry now. 'I should have been with him. For the abseiling and the scavenger hunt. The only thing I've done with him properly was that sandcastle competition. I feel like I've let him down completely.'

'You haven't let him down at all,' Maya said. 'He's had a great time, Eli—and you gave him the freedom to let him try things he's never been allowed to do before. Like the pony riding. And the abseiling. He's loved everything he's done here. He knew you'd see the photos of him on that cliff and be proud of him. He knows how much you love him. It's me that's the problem. He doesn't want to share you.' She caught her breath. 'It's because of me he's run away, isn't it? Because of…*us*…'

The answer to her question was in his eyes. There was something like an apology there as well. Because, even if he did still love her, he would never do anything that could harm Simon in any way. Maya got that. She wouldn't allow Simon to be hurt either. She cared deeply about every child she met at camp but this one was also the son of the man she loved and that took her concern to a whole new, agonising level.

Eli gave a single nod, as if he agreed with her unspoken thought.

'I think you might be right,' he said aloud.

Maya's heart sank even further. This felt like the final blow to any dream she might have had about them being together again. Or the three of them becoming a family.

But Eli was, apparently, agreeing to something else.

'He could have been thinking about that damn flower all evening. Where was it growing? Where is that cliff, exactly?'

'It's part of the headland at the end of the lagoon beach. We need to check the beach anyway so we can go and have a look.'

They made their way to the beach, the light from the powerful torches on their hard hats bouncing as they ran. Eli had a first aid pack on his back that they'd taken from the trailer as they'd left the medical centre and Maya had a heavy coil of rope looped over her shoulder. She sent up a silent prayer that any loose coconuts had already been blown from the trees in the first hours of this storm as they went under the crescent of palm trees that framed the lagoon beach.

The beach couldn't have been any different to her first day at camp this year. The day she'd seen Eli again for the first time after so many years. She'd been walking down here at daybreak with the wind no more than a delightful tropical breeze and the only waves way out on the reef. She'd had no idea what lay ahead of her when Mike had told her that he'd scored the perfect member for their medical team at this year's camp—an emergency medicine consultant who had a special interest in paediatrics. Someone who'd been persuaded to come because his son qualified to be a camp attendee due to his Type A haemophilia. When she'd had no idea that she was about to find herself face to face with the man she'd loved so much and then lost so long ago.

Now, it felt as if her entire world was a very different place, emotionally as well as physically. The wind was still strong enough to make it hard to stay upright and there were waves that were coming so far up the beach from the lagoon that Maya had to jump out of the way of the foam. She stumbled then, on a coconut perhaps or a piece of driftwood, or maybe it was the gust of wind that made her lose her balance and fall. Eli's gesture to hold out his hand and help her up was automatic but he didn't let go of it as they ran along the beach and the squeeze on her heart was just as powerful as the wind.

'Simon...' Maya cupped one hand to her mouth and called again. '*Si*-mon...'

They kept shouting for Simon, although they both knew that even if he was really close he wouldn't hear them. Was the thought that he might hear them—and call back—the real reason for doing it? Because it gave them hope?

'*Si*-mon...' Eli's voice was getting a bit hoarse. 'Where are you?'

They were at the end of the beach now. The tumble of rocks was directly in front of them but Maya knew the track that would take them higher, through trees and shrubs to the side of the rocks and onto the wide ledge that provided such a good base for the cliff they used for their beginner abseiling sessions.

Simon had thought he'd seen a ginger plant growing on the path that continued up the steep slope, on the other side of the ledge, that they used to get to the top of the cliff and then abseil down. In daylight, the start of that path also provided a view down to the next bay past the lagoon. This was a beach that was open to the sea and it had waves so it was used for teaching children who wanted to learn to surf or bodyboard. Maya couldn't see the beach but she could hear waves that were big enough to be crashing onto the foot of the rocky outcrop that formed the barrier between this beach and the resort's lagoon.

Looking down made the beam of light from the torch on Maya's helmet catch the spray from a wave that was reaching high enough to be metres above the hidden beach and it looked thick enough to mimic a snowstorm. If a storm surge made the waves any higher than they were right now, this ledge that they used for the abseiling would be in danger of being undermined and possibly washed away. The edges already looked dodgy...

'Oh, my God...' Maya froze.

'What?' Eli was right behind her. The additional strength of his torchlight made what Maya was looking at even clearer. A small figure clinging onto the rocks below the ledge. The sky-blue camp tee shirt with the yellow circle and the palm tree on the front. A pale, terrified face was looking up at them, but Simon was trying to shield his eyes from the bright light.

The sound Eli made was almost a growl. He tried to step past Maya and get out onto the ledge but she put her arm out to stop him.

'No—' Her tone was urgent.

Her body was awash with adrenaline and it made her thoughts go so fast she could barely catch them.

The thought of Eli going onto that ledge and having it crumble—of him falling onto the rocks and hitting his head or, worse, losing him for ever because he'd been washed into a vicious sea was unbelievably horrific.

Dear Lord…had this been how Eli felt whenever she'd done something challenging enough to be risky? Did he have to fight feeling like that every time he let Simon do something that might not be absolutely safe—like going on a climbing wall? She'd had *no* idea how overwhelming it could be.

The thoughts were there and then gone in the space of a blink.

'You can't go anywhere near the edge, Eli.'

Her words were even more of a command than Mike had given him to make sure he wasn't out here alone. 'You're too heavy. You'd end up down on the rocks. Or in the sea.' She tried to aim her torch at Simon's feet rather than directly into his face. 'Simon?' She shouted as loudly as she could, after a wave had broken and before the next could start. 'Can you hear me, sweetheart?'

She could see him nod his head in the edge of the beam of light.

'I'm coming down to get you, okay?'

'No…' Eli sounded distraught. 'I can't just stay here and do nothing.'

'You won't be doing nothing.' Maya was uncoiling the rope she'd been carrying. 'I want you at the back of the ledge, right beside the cliff. Don't go anywhere near the edge. You're going to hold the end of this rope after I find a rock to wrap it around.'

'It's not enough. I need to—'

Maya cut him off. 'This is *the* most important thing you *can* do,' she told him fiercely. 'Just being there, holding on, will be what it takes to keep both of us safe.'

A rope around her waist was nothing like as safe as wearing a harness but it was better than nothing. Maya went over the edge of this flat ledge, well away from being above Simon, knowing that she could be dislodging a shower of small rocks and dirt. She got down to the top of a huge boulder and then stopped to look around in the hope of finding a way down to the next step in this outcrop but, without the proper gear and safety measures, there was nothing she could see that was anywhere near safe enough to try. She looped the rope around a jagged cone of rock and lay down on her stomach to look over the much rounder top of this weathered boulder. She was so much closer to Simon. If she stretched out her arm, she could almost touch him.

But it wasn't close enough.

'It's okay,' she called out. 'I'm going to get you out of here. Are you hurt?'

It looked as if Simon was crying. He said something that Maya couldn't hear but, even though he was clearly terrified, he was listening. He pushed himself to stand up so, if he *was* hurt, at least it wasn't badly enough to stop him being able to move.

'Can you do something for me, Si?' Maya didn't wait for an answer. 'Do you remember that day you first did the climbing wall?'

His nod was dubious.

'Can you see the lump of rock just in front of you? Like a step?'

He was looking in the right direction.

'And just above your shoulder, there's another rock. Can you put your foot on the step and reach up for that rock with your hand?'

Slowly, Simon followed the instructions she was shouting. Maya held her breath. She tried not to imagine how dangerous a gust of wind or a sudden shower of sea spray could be. It seemed as if the wind had dropped, but who knew how long that could last?

'Good job,' she told Simon. 'It's just like the climbing wall. There's another bit that's going to be just right for a step, but don't let go with your hands just yet. I'll shine my torch on where your foot needs to go.'

Simon was hesitating.

'You can do this,' she called. 'Pretend it's the climbing wall, Si, and your dad's watching you. And...' Maya could feel her heart breaking a little '...he's *so* proud of you...'

Yes... Simon was moving sideways. Feeling for the foothold. Getting closer.

'Let go with your left hand and reach up.' Maya was leaning down as far as she could. 'Catch my hand...'

There was a split second where Simon seemed to hang in space and then Maya felt the touch of his fingers and slid her hand past them to wrap around his wrist. He felt so light as she pulled him up. So fragile. So precious. She wriggled them both back from the edge of the boulder so that she could wrap her arms around him. The wind and rain and crashing surf beneath them became almost irrelevant as she focused for just a breath or two on trying to offer this child some warmth. And love. Trying to make him feel safe.

'Does anything hurt?'

Simon was shivering too hard to speak. But he was hanging on to her with a grip that was strong enough to let her know it was safe to try and get them both back to the ledge.

'Don't let go,' she said against his ear. 'Dad's waiting for us. Just up here…'

It had probably only taken five minutes from when Eli had positioned himself beside the cliff to be the anchor on the rope to when he saw Maya and Simon climb back onto the ledge but it had felt like the longest period of time he'd ever had to survive. It was only when his lungs started burning that he remembered to stop holding his breath and fill them with oxygen again.

Maya was putting her life on the line to save his son. He was so afraid for her but so incredibly proud of her at the same time. This was who she was and he wouldn't want to change a thing about this woman he loved so much.

He was so afraid for Simon, too.

And…he was afraid for himself. Because how could he go on without either of the people he loved this much in his life? Nothing would ever feel complete. He would never feel whole.

The moment when he saw them appear almost undid him. When he could let go of the rope and scoop Simon into his arms he had no idea what percentage of the rain running down his face was actually tears. He held Simon close with one arm and used his other arm to bring Maya closer.

He held them tightly. He'd never felt this relieved in his life. This grateful. He never wanted to let either of them go. Ever. And yet hadn't he just realised that he would never want to change a thing about what made Maya the person she was? Trying too hard to protect the people he loved carried the risk of stopping them being who they wanted to be. Who they really were.

It was a moment of astonishing clarity. The way he was feeling in this moment, as if every one of his senses was at maximum capacity, was like nothing he'd ever felt before.

He could feel the warmth of the bodies so close to his own and the chill of the dying wind around them. He could smell, and taste, the sea spray in the air. He could hear the sniffle of Simon trying not to cry and, was it his imagination or could he see—in Maya's eyes—a depth of love that made his heart feel as if it was about to explode?

Was this simply the joy of being alive?

Was the flip side of extreme fear an exhilaration like no other?

And had he, in fact, been stopping himself from being the person *he* really was because he'd given fear too much power? Had his anxiety about the safety of the people he cared most about become a kind of white noise that was stopping him from being able to feel what it was like to be really alive?

To feel like *this*?

Not being able to feel every nuance of the best that life could offer was too high a price to pay for not having to feel the worst that could—but might actually never—happen.

There was a new message in Maya's eyes now. They needed to get back to shelter. Back to the medical centre where they could make sure Simon was really safe. Eli could feel him shivering and being too cold, on top of being on the flip side of feeling far too frightened, could easily be masking the signs and symptoms of injury.

'Let's go,' he said, matching his words with movement.

Simon's head jerked up. 'Maya's coming too, isn't she?'

'She sure is.' Eli hadn't quite broken that eye contact with Maya. 'She's showing us the way.'

CHAPTER ELEVEN

WRAPPED IN THE foil survival blanket from the first aid kit, Simon looked as if he had fallen asleep in his father's arms by the time they got back to the medical centre. Mike had the treatment room ready and well heated.

'I've got a bucket of ice from the kitchens,' he told Eli. 'And the storm's definitely blowing through. If we need to get Simon to the main island for imaging we can't do here, we should be able to have the helicopter available by midday.'

But that was still hours away and Maya knew how worried Eli had to be. She felt sick with worry herself.

'Your Factor VIII supplies are in the fridge here, aren't they?'

'Yes. Could you find the testing kit, please, Maya? It looks like a blood glucose monitoring kit.'

He was putting Simon down gently onto the bed and, to her relief, she saw that he was looking more awake, but she knew that a head injury and brain bleed was the most serious injury someone with haemophilia could suffer. It could be fatal.

Eli wasn't showing any sign of the stress he had to be under, however. He was so warm and reassuring with Simon that Maya was starting to believe that everything was going to be okay.

Everything.

Even whatever was going to happen—or not happen—between herself and Eli?

She handed the small, zipped pouch to Eli and then helped position the pillows and tuck warm blankets around Simon. He pricked the end of one of Simon's fingers and collected the drop of blood onto the test strip.

'This will let us know what level of Factor VIII he's got on board but we'll need to start an infusion if there's any sign of injury. We'll need to get his levels to at least fifty percent of normal in that case.'

'I didn't know you could do a finger prick test for Factor VIII.'

'And thrombin on this one. We're part of an international trial for home testing monitors. The technology is getting more reliable all the time.' Eli put the test meter down and shone a pen torch across Simon's eyes, to check pupil sizes and reactions.

'Did you get knocked out?' he asked.

'No. I remember everything. I dropped my torch and it rolled over the edge and when I tried to see where it had gone, a big bit of dirt broke off. I was kind of sitting on it as we went down.'

'Like a surfboard?' Maya asked. 'That was a smart move, Si.'

Not that it had been intentional, of course, but the cushioning could well have saved him from far more serious injuries.

'So you didn't hit your head at all?' Eli's fingers were in the damp spikes of Simon's hair that had been quickly towel dried to try and help warm him up. Maya could almost feel that gentle touch herself.

'I don't think so.'

'Does anything hurt anywhere else? Can you take a deep breath?'

Simon pulled in a huge breath. 'My tummy kind of hurts. And my elbow...'

Maya was careful not to let her expression change. Internal bleeding was another big thing to worry about. And bleeding into a joint could have lasting effects on movement and function.

She watched Eli unwrap the blankets around Simon and help take his shorts off. As he passed them to Maya, something fell out of the pocket. Something red.

'Oh—' she exclaimed, stooping to pick up the long, and very squashed, bloom. 'You did find a ginger flower, Si. You'll be the only person who found everything for the scavenger hunt.'

'I didn't get it for that,' he said. 'Ow…that hurts, Dad.'

'Sorry, buddy. You've got a big bruise coming up on your hip.'

Was the blood below his skin there coming from an internal injury—like trauma to his liver?

Eli flattened his hand and pressed gently on the different quadrants of Simon's abdomen. 'Tell me if anything hurts,' he instructed.

Maya could see that familiar vertical line of concentration on Eli's face. She wanted to distract Simon in case he interpreted it as concern that his father was finding something seriously wrong with him.

'You did so well, climbing up off those rocks,' she told him. 'You remembered everything you learned on the climbing wall, didn't you?'

'It was scary,' Simon confessed.

'Of course it was.' Maya nodded. 'But you were really brave.'

'I'm glad I didn't lose the flower.'

Maya shook her head. 'Why did you go looking for it, if it wasn't to finish off your scavenger basket?'

His eyes looked too big in a very pale face. 'I wanted to find it for you,' he said.

'For *me*?'

'Ana said it was a special flower because it got used when people get married in Fiji. And you said it was one of your favourite flowers.'

'It is. I love that you wanted to get me one, but...' Maya's gaze flew to Eli's. Was this another reason why she could blame herself for Simon hurting himself?

Eli's glance told her not to.

'You shouldn't have gone out in the storm, Si,' he said. 'You know that, don't you?'

'Yes.' Simon's voice was small. 'I'm sorry, Dad...'

'I know...' Eli touched his son's face. 'I'm sorry, too. I should have been there to take care of you.'

But Simon shook his head. 'You were taking care of other people and that's your job. I'm not a little kid any more. I *can* take care of myself.'

'I know you can.' Eli smoothed the spikes of hair off Simon's forehead. 'And you don't ever need to collect any special prizes, you know. I couldn't be more proud of you than I already am.'

It felt like a very private moment between a father and his son. It was enough to create a lump in Maya's throat that felt far too big to swallow.

Eli looked like he was blinking back a tear himself as he shifted his gaze to Mike. 'Can we get a cold pack to go on that bruised hip?'

'Coming right up.'

Eli moved on with this rapid but thorough initial survey.

'We'll need one for this elbow, too. And a compression bandage.'

Mike had started bandaging the bruised elbow as Eli got ready to set up an infusion. The only other finding had been found a bumped knee that was painful to bend, which would need the same treatment of rest, ice, compression and elevation. With all vital sign measurements stable and normal enough to suggest that Simon had somehow avoided an injury that could be causing serious, unseen internal bleeding, the level of tension in the room was beginning to decrease noticeably.

An hour later, with better levels of Factor VIII, thanks to the infusion, some pain relief and being tucked up in a warm, comfortable bed, all Simon wanted to do was to go to sleep and his eyes were drifting shut.

Mike was back with Ma'afu and Tevita. Danny and James, the helicopter pilots, were in the office, getting updates on the improving weather conditions and planning the first flights to evacuate their patients as soon as they were given clearance.

The first fingers of light in a murky dawn

could be seen through the high windows of the treatment room.

'I'll have to go back to the village soon,' Maya told Eli. 'I promised I would.'

'I'll stay with Simon. It's time I refreshed those cold packs on his bruising and I want to check his Factor VIII levels again.'

Maya was trying to make her feet move and take her towards the door but they weren't co-operating.

She wanted to stay with Simon as well. To watch him like a hawk for any sign of his condition deteriorating. To be near Eli because she knew how much of his concern he was keeping carefully hidden.

No…actually, she just wanted to be near Eli.

Taking this step away from him now might be the first of countless steps that would see them on the opposite sides of the world again.

In the end, it was Eli that took a step.

Towards her.

He held out his arms and Maya went into them without hesitation. She felt them wrap around her and pull her close. She could hear—and feel—Eli's heart beating.

'I haven't said thank you,' he said. 'It was you who got him off those rocks. If the tide had come up any further…' His voice trailed off and Maya felt a shudder ripple through his body.

'I couldn't have done it by myself,' Maya said. 'It was Simon who was brave enough to close the distance between us so that I could get hold of him and it wasn't an easy thing to do. He had to find footholds and handholds and make himself move even though he didn't have any safety gear on at all.'

She could feel Eli taking in a deep breath. 'You told me, that day when Simon got into your session at the climbing wall, that it would be better for him to learn how to do something like that safely than to put himself in real danger by trying it when no one was watching. It was only because of you teaching him what to do that he could help get himself off those rocks. You saved his life, Maya. And mine… I would have gone after him if you hadn't stopped me and I wouldn't have known how to do that safely.'

Maya's smile was shaky. 'Maybe you should come to a climbing wall session yourself.'

'Maybe I will. Next time we're here.'

'Are we coming back again, Dad?'

Maya gasped, stepping hurriedly away from Eli, turning towards the bed to find Simon watching them both, his eyes wide open.

'Um…yes, I hope so,' Eli said. 'That is, if you'd like to come back, Si.'

Simon nodded. 'I want to come back. But I'd quite like to go home again, too.'

'We'll go home very soon,' Eli told him. He perched on the side of the bed. 'I need to take you to the hospital and make absolutely sure you're okay. Camp Reki's due to finish soon, anyway.'

'I want to go to Australia, too,' Simon added.

'Really?' Eli sounded cautious. 'For a holiday?'

Simon didn't answer his father. 'Are you going back to Australia, Maya?' he asked.

'Yes. That's where I live.'

'But you used to live in New Zealand.'

'Yes.'

'That's where you lived, isn't it, Dad? When I was a baby?'

'Yes. I've told you that story.' Eli reached out to stroke Simon's hair. 'How I heard about the terrible accident your mum had and I jumped on a plane and came back to England so I could look after you.'

'Did you live with Maya? Because she was your girlfriend?'

Maya could see Eli taking a deep breath. He'd told her he had always been honest with Simon.

'Yes, I did.'

'So why did you leave her behind?'

Maya's eyes widened. So did Eli's. He opened his mouth and then closed it again.

'You told me you'd never leave someone you really loved behind. And…'

Simon was frowning quite fiercely and it reminded Maya of the way Eli looked when he was totally focused on something very important.

'And you really love Maya, don't you?'

'I do.' Eli looked from Simon to Maya. 'I do,' he repeated softly. Solemnly.

She could see the truth of that in his eyes—the glow that was warming her entire body. 'I don't think I ever stopped loving you, Maya.'

Eli's gaze was back on Simon. 'But I love you, too, Si. I always will. That's never, ever going to change, okay?'

Simon ignored that question, too.

'And you love Dad, don't you, Maya?'

'I do,' Maya said. She waited for Eli's gaze to catch her own again. 'I never stopped loving you either.'

'That's why I went to find your favourite flower,' Simon said. 'I wanted you to love *me*, too.'

'Oh, Simon…' Maya went to sit on the other side of the bed so she could hug Simon. Gently, taking care not to bump his bruises. 'You don't have to give me flowers, sweetheart. I *do* love you already.'

'So…' Simon was stifling a huge yawn as he

turned to his father again. 'Does that mean I'm going to have a mum *and* a dad?'

Eli caught Maya's gaze over the top of Simon's head. 'I hope so,' he said softly.

Maya couldn't say anything. The words were caught somewhere in her chest but she didn't need to say anything aloud, did she? She could tell Eli just how much she also hoped that was going to happen just by holding that gaze.

And smiling.

They *were* going to find a way to be together. They were going to become a family.

'There's no rush,' Eli added. 'It's a big thing for you to get used to, Si. It's a big thing for us, too. Maybe we'll have that holiday in Australia first.'

'And then we'll come back here.' Simon's eyes were drifting shut again. 'For another camp.'

'We will.'

'And you can get married here.'

'Maybe...'

'Ana says that some people who get married here like to carry a whole bunch of ginger flowers.' Simon's words were getting quieter. 'I might need to find some more...'

He was sound asleep a moment later.

Eli was smiling at Maya. 'Would you like that?'

'A bunch of ginger flowers?' Maya was teasing him. 'Yes, I would. They're one of my favourite flowers, you know.'

'And the rest?' Eli's smile faded. 'I love you, Maya. I need you in my life. Simon needs you in *his* life. I want to marry you this time. To be with you. For ever.'

This was serious. He was asking about the rest of her life. The rest of *their* lives.

'Oh, yes.' Maya's tone was just as serious. She had no doubt about this at all. 'I can't think of anything I'd like more…'

EPILOGUE

Three years later...

IT WAS THE first night of Camp Reki.

Bonfire night.

S'mores night.

Maya was sitting on the edge of the circle surrounding a bonfire that had burnt down enough to be no more than a pile of embers. Camp staff and caregivers were helping children roast marshmallows on long sticks. There were smiles and laughter everywhere but Maya saw a dismayed expression on one young girl's face as her marshmallow burst into flames, slipped off her stick and fell onto the hot coals. Her carer looked just as disappointed but, before the girl could burst into tears, someone was there to rescue her.

Eli was there. He'd been about to start toasting the marshmallows on his own stick but he'd witnessed the disaster and crouched beside her to not only put a fresh marshmallow on her stick but to show her how to turn it and take it away from the heat before disaster struck again. She had a smile on her face in no time at all.

Maya was smiling as well.

Every day she thought she couldn't love Eli Peters any more than she did already.

And every day she proved herself wrong and she could feel her heart softening enough to get that little bit bigger so it could hold that extra bit of love.

If he wasn't surprising her with what a caring husband and father he was, she could be blown away by his devotion to his work and the concern he had for every person who came under his care. Okay, he still worried too much sometimes but that was just because he cared so much.

She had married a kind man.

They would be celebrating their second anniversary during this year's camp. How many people were lucky enough to be able to celebrate every year in the actual place that both their wedding and honeymoon had taken place?

In a tropical island paradise?

It had been the most perfect day in her life.

Everybody at camp—and in the village—had been invited. Maya had worn a long, floaty white dress, frangipani flowers in her hair and she had a huge bunch of bright red ginger flowers in her hands.

Picked by Simon, of course. And his mate Carlos.

They'd both been online to find out why the colour red was important for weddings.

'It's special all over the world,' Simon had announced. *'It brings good luck for a happy and harmonious marriage—whatever harmonious means.'*

'It's a good thing,' Maya had assured him.

'Apparently it represents love, power, passion and fertility,' Carlos had added. He'd winked at Maya. *'That's a good thing, too, yeah?'*

Maya had simply winked back at him.

They'd been married at sunset, barefoot on the lagoon beach, under an archway of hibiscus flowers that looked like fragments of the sky's colour as the sun slowly sank. Simon and Carlos had been Eli's groomsmen. Ana and Hazel had been Maya's bridesmaids. The party afterwards had been epic, with island music, singing and dancing, an absolute feast of delicious food. And s'mores for dessert. Because it was camp, after all.

Where Maya and Eli had been so unexpectedly reunited after so many years apart.

Where they'd chosen to make public their commitment to each other that would last for the rest of their lives.

Where they fully intended to return every

year, not only to celebrate but to be a part of Camp Reki.

The s'mores had been Simon's idea but both Maya and Eli had been more than happy to embrace it.

Because it hadn't been simply a ceremony between two people, had it? It had been the formal recognition of the family they had created. They'd moved, as a family, to live in Australia. They lived near a beach in Sydney, Eli was in charge of an emergency department that was even busier than where he'd been in London and Simon was thriving in his new country and school, embracing every new adventure that came his way.

Maya scanned the crowd around the bonfire, wondering where Simon had got to but not at all worried that she couldn't see him. He was twelve years old now, going on thirteen, although she and Eli often joked that it was more like he was going on thirty because he was so grown-up and responsible.

He looked after his own Factor VIII infusions now and knew what to do if he had any bleeding episodes. He also made his own decisions about how to keep himself safe enough to enjoy his new passions of surfing and scrambling up indoor climbing walls. Between having his own fun at camp this year with other activities, he was going to be taking Maya's place to help teach the younger children about the challenges and fun of climbing.

Right now, though, he would be with his friends, which was exactly where he should be. What tweenager wanted to hang out all the time with their parents? Maybe Tevita had given him a drum and he was part of the group providing the music this evening that would always take Maya straight back to the joy of her wedding.

A joy that had never gone away but had an intensity here, on the island, that made it feel brand-new all over again.

Maya's gaze sought out Eli and she saw that he was busy toasting his own marshmallows. He'd go to the long table next and get the crackers and chocolate and then he'd bring the treat to where she was sitting. Maya licked her lips. She couldn't wait…

'You look happy.'

Maya turned her head and her smile widened. 'Hey, Mike.' She nodded. 'I couldn't be happier.'

'Happy anniversary.'

'Thank you. It's going to be the best one yet. I was just thinking how lucky we are to be able to come back here to celebrate every year. Especially when I'm not even here in an official capacity this time.'

'Wouldn't be Camp Reki these days without

the Peters family,' Mike said. 'I see Eli's getting your anniversary dessert ready.'

'Yes. Maybe I should go and find Simon.'

'He's with Tevita, helping him entertain his wee nephew while Ana's busy with the camp kids.' He grinned. 'Getting in a bit of practice, I reckon. Did you hear that Alice's parents are coming to visit this week? And her brother, Jake?'

'I did.' Maya's smile was poignant. Alice would always be part of her own story. *Their* stories. Hers and Eli's.

Mike's smile mirrored hers. 'They wanted to be here when we unveil the memorial for Alice. They also want Carlos to meet Jake.'

'Oh? Why?'

'They asked if they could do something more than put up a memorial here. I told them about the trust fund that's there to help kids who can't afford to get to camp on their own. I also told them I'm planning to help Carlos if he doesn't get a scholarship. And I told them that helping kids like Alice was why he decided he wanted to go to medical school. They want to make a significant contribution to the trust fund. And Jake wants to encourage Carlos to achieve his dreams. It could be the start of a lifelong friendship.' Mike let his breath out in a sigh. 'That's what camp is all about, really, isn't it? Making lifelong friends?'

'And making dreams come true,' Maya agreed. She could see Eli coming towards her now, with the s'mores on a paper plate. 'It certainly worked for me.'

Mike just smiled again. He lifted a hand in greeting to Eli but then faded into the crowd to carry on with his usual goal of spending time with every camp attendee on the first evening.

Eli sat down beside Maya.

'Better have one of these fast,' he warned. 'Simon's on his way.'

Maya laughed. 'He must have been keeping a close eye on you. He does love s'mores.'

She picked one of the cracker sandwiches and bit into the sticky, chocolatey, sweet and salty treat.

'Mmm…' she said with her mouth full. 'So do I.' She grinned at Eli. 'I think it's my new craving.'

Eli laughed, putting his hand on the impressive bump of Maya's belly. For a long moment, it was simply a moment between them. An exchange of a look that spoke of limitless love. Of gratitude for everything they had and the excitement for what was coming. It was also a look of pure happiness.

'You are eating for three,' Eli said. He pushed

himself back to his feet. 'I'd better go and make...' he rolled his eyes to warn of a bad joke '...s'more?'

Simon was right behind him and he thought it was hilarious. 'S'more s'mores,' he said. 'Good one, Dad.'

'Come and help me make then,' Eli said, putting his arm over Simon's shoulders. 'Those ones are just for Mum. They're her new craving.'

Maya watched the two of them walking back towards the dying fire but, as if they'd been reading each other's minds, they both looked over their shoulders at exactly the same time and smiled at her.

She smiled back, of course. But she suddenly found herself blinking back tears.

Happy tears.

She could feel the babies moving inside her. Two girls who were due to arrive in a couple of months.

The Peters family was growing.

And there it was again. That feeling of her heart expanding to accommodate even more love. Maya had thought she'd been perfectly truthful when she'd told Mike that she couldn't be happier.

But clearly there was still more to come...

* * * * *

If you enjoyed this story,
check out these other great reads from
Alison Roberts

City Vet, Country Temptation
Falling for Her Forbidden Flatmate
Miracle Twins to Heal Them
Therapy Pup to Heal the Surgeon

All available now!

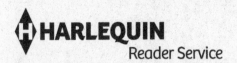
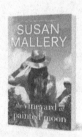
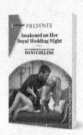
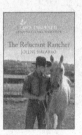
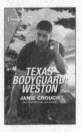